WHAT OTHE~~RS AR~~
A CAREGIVER'S GU~~IDE TO THROAT CANCER ...~~

"This Guide is excellent, and I would highly recommend it to anyone who shares a diagnosis of throat cancer or has a loved one who does. I am grateful to Susan Grant for filling this niche and recommend this book as a guide through the day-by-day challenges that are not generally addressed by standard medical care. I am very impressed with its thoroughness."

— *Gregory E. Keyes, M.D.*

"I love this book. A person going through cancer treatment and their caretakers are going through a tough, hard time. Any gesture of warmth or kindness can be hard to find and greatly appreciated. I feel this book provides not only excellent practical information and delicious recipes, but most importantly, the heart of Susan Grant can be felt on every page. Bravo Susan! Well done."

—*Saari Sedillo, Patient Advocate & Alternative Healthcare Provider*

"This book will serve as an anchor, a reference, and a lifeline during the treatment of any head and neck cancer. Down-to-earth advice from someone who has been there and back".

—*Annie Murphy, M.D. and Medical Oncologist*

A CAREGIVER'S GUIDE TO THROAT CANCER

Honesty, hope, and humor
to help you navigate the wild ride called Throat Cancer!

Susan Grant

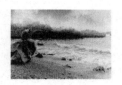

Bella Vista Publishing
"Perspective is everything!"

www.BellaVistaPublishing.com

DISCLAIMER
This book was written for the purpose of providing helpful information on the topics discussed herein. Any opinions or ideas expressed in this book represent the personal experiences and viewpoints of the author. The ideas and suggestions in this book are not meant to be a substitute for the advice and treatment provided by your physician.

Neither the author nor the publisher is providing medical, health, or any other kind of personal professional services or advice to those who are reading this book, nor are they liable or responsible for any losses, damages, or injuries allegedly arising from any information or suggestions contained in this book. Neither the publisher nor author is responsible for your specific allergy or health requirements, or for any adverse or allergic reactions to the recipes or suggestions in this book.

Published by Bella Vista Publishing: www.BellaVistaPublishing.com

Library of Congress Control Number: 2012940885

ISBN 978-0-9852179-3-6
eBook ISBN 978-0-9852179-3-8

Manufactured in the United States of America

For those of you who need a little guidance,
peace of mind, and humor
amidst the unexpected fear and chaos
that cancer brings.
There is light at the end of the tunnel,
and it is not an oncoming train!

Remember to laugh, love, and enjoy your life,
no matter what cards you've been dealt.
Listen quietly. Look deeply.
Little miracles are everywhere.

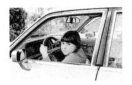

Table of Contents

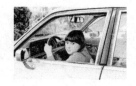

Acknowledgements

Many thanks to all the wonderfully supportive friends and family who were there for us throughout the whole cancer treatment and recovery process, including: Mary Pizzo, Beth Goodnough, Carl Barenboim, Jackie Pizzo, Tricia Lord, Lorilee Houston, Vera Williams, Kalie Rae, The Barenboim clan (*Leesa, Elaine, and Herm*), and Bob Haslanger. A round of applause to all those who contributed both personally and anonymously to our Cancer Recovery Fund. You made our burdens lighter, our days brighter, and helped keep us afloat during the most difficult time of our lives. We couldn't have made it through without you. A grateful hug and huge thank you to our expert and reassuring oncology support team led by Dr. Ann E. Murphy and the radiation oncology team led by Dr. Berit Madsen at Peninsula Cancer Center. Quite frankly, you saved my husband's life and got us to laugh a bit in the process. This is a rare talent! Many thanks as well to Dr. Gregory Keyes who was always there for us whenever we needed him (*even on Sundays!*). And last, but not least, a tummy rub and an endless supply of favorite cookies to my two little dogs, Bella and Madame Boo Boo, who not only kept us entertained and charmed with their adorable antics, but also managed to cheer up many distraught patients in the waiting room.

Chapter 1

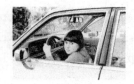

Why I Wrote This Book

This is the book I wish I had been given when I suddenly learned my husband had Stage IV Throat Cancer. We didn't have a clue what to expect or what to do and we were being whisked into the medical system right away. We needed help! Like a tourist traveling in a foreign land, I needed a guidebook - in plain English - to help me navigate the muddy and often confusing road of throat cancer - and to help my husband and myself successfully make it through the whole ordeal.

Quite simply, there wasn't a book like this available - and I sure wanted one. I had hoped the doctors would hand us a booklet filled with ideas, suggestions, shopping lists, recipes, etc., but no such luck. When I suggested to the clinic that a booklet of this nature was needed, they thought it was a great idea. So here it is!

It was during my husband's cancer treatments and all the difficulties and successes we experienced, that I decided to write this book. No need for you to reinvent the wheel. Whether you are a patient, a caring family member, a friend of the patient, or a caregiver - my hope is that our experience, advice, wisdom, and humor will make your journey a little easier and your path a little smoother. Help is on the way!

This book is meant to be in addition to - and not a substitute for - the medical advice and treatment you will receive from your oncologists. I wrote this book to help you in the way that I needed help most:

- To get the big picture of what to expect from throat cancer treatments and procedures along with a brief discussion about the ever-changing symptoms of throat cancer.

- To make sure you have the tools, equipment, supplies, and resources you'll need at home and on the road.

- To help you understand and manage your mountain of medical bills.

- To help you learn what you can do to keep your loved one as comfortable, healthy, and pain-free as possible.

- To give you advice on how to create the simplest, healthiest, most enjoyable, and nutritious food to support healing.

- To give you some tips and tools to stay centered and sane while surviving the whole cancer ordeal - and maybe even find some humor in the process.

- And more...

Please bear in mind that these suggestions and ideas are from my own personal experience based on what worked for us. I am happy to share them with you. While I am not a doctor, I've had many years of experience using nutrition and other modalities for healing. I also have *"the chip"* for organizing, streamlining, and doing whatever I can to make things work from the inside out. Had it not been for my innate skills in this regard, we could not have weathered the whole cancer process as well as we did.

There is hope for you and your loved one. At this writing, it has been over a year since my husband finished his throat cancer treatments. His recent P.E.T. scan revealed he is cancer-free and his doctors told us that he won't need any more scans. This is great news - and something to celebrate! So my advice is this: get educated, stay the course, keep a positive attitude, do what you can to support the healing process, and hopefully, you'll have something to celebrate a year from now, too!

Wishing you all the best on your journey!

Chapter 2

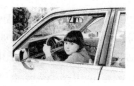

Introduction

About our personal story ...

This was to be my year for a sabbatical. After 15 plus years as a professional photographer doing weddings and portraits, it was time for a break and a fresh start. As an artist, I'm always inventing things - and this was going to be my year to create something new. Maybe even write a book. Little did I know that in clearing my calendar and my life for something new I would also be creating the time and energy to care for my husband when he needed me most. I couldn't have written the script any better than that. We'd just moved to a beautiful house surrounded by nature, which proved to be the perfect healing sanctuary for both of us.

For about six months, my husband, John had been complaining of a sore throat and earache that came and went. Every so often he'd go for another checkup and was always told the same thing: *"We can't find anything wrong with you."* I was very concerned. John was not his usual energetic self. While he was not debilitated enough to stop working, my husband was exhausted and in pain. When he began losing weight fairly rapidly, I got scared. Happy to have started losing *"his little paunch,"* John thought nothing of it. But I thought something was terribly wrong. One of his doctors began treating him for a salivary infection, as my husband was all puffed out like an

"Amazonian frog" just below his chin on one side. The antibiotics seemed to be working. Not entirely, but mostly. So we asked for an extension to his antibiotics. But it never fully cleared up. At that point we decided to see a well-respected ENT (Ear, Nose, and Throat Doctor) in Seattle, and that's when all the fun began.

We honestly thought the ENT would do a few scans and determine it was an allergy or an infection and simply prescribe a new medication that would work like a charm. No such luck. After a few scans, the ENT scheduled what he jokingly called a *"little procedure"* and wouldn't tell us what he was looking for. I pushed and prodded the ENT to tell me what was going on, and at first he joked, *"I'm going to take a big mallet and hit your husband on the head."* We did not find this amusing. But he finally admitted he was going to perform a biopsy in my husband's throat. He wouldn't tell us why. We went along with it, but honestly had no idea what was going on. Everything was happening so fast …

For many reasons, our big biopsy adventure was quite an unpleasant ordeal, as we seemed to slip through the cracks at every turn. Even reputable doctors and hospitals have their problems - and we seemed to be subjected to quite a few of them, which compounded the stress we were already under.

During the biopsy, the ENT discovered a large tumor in my husband's throat, which had not yet spread to the lungs, but did involve a few of his lymph nodes. It was Squamous Cell Carcinoma. For some unknown reason, the ENT did not tell my husband or me what he'd discovered during the operation. In fact, he told me specifically he was unsure what was wrong with my husband but insisted he would need to take more (*expensive*) tests. Only when my husband refused to take more tests did the ENT admit what he found. We were unprepared for the diagnosis and did not know what to expect. We were frightened and vulnerable. The ENT tried to rush us to sign up with his oncology team, but we weren't signing up for anything immediately. We were unhappy with the services we received at his clinic and wanted to find a team that would better serve our needs closer to home.

Fortunately, one of my husband's dear friends recommended a wonderful oncologist in our area who really understood my husband's condition as well as the newest and best protocols to get him well. She was kind, caring, forthright, and reassuring. Without hesitation, we chose her to set up and oversee my husband's treatment regime. Her clinic specialized in chemotherapy, which was to be administered once a week. The other part of the treatment was radiation, which she set up and coordinated with a state-of-the-art radiation oncology center nearby. Radiation treatments involved intensive 20-minute sessions five days a week for 7 weeks. A brutal, but doable schedule.

To our relief the doctors were talking *"cure."* They told us that in many cases, throat cancer is curable and they believed my husband's cancer was one of them. This gave us hope. But then came the shock. John had always been the strong one in our relationship. My rock. He was usually healthy with boundless energy. Maybe an occasional headache or bout of allergies, but rarely even a cold. John wasn't a smoker or much of a drinker. Just an occasional glass of wine or beer with dinner. For the 20 years we'd been together we lived a pretty clean, healthy life. And, because of my own health issues, we ate mostly organic foods, lived in rural places where pollution was minimal, and used natural, healthy, chemical-free products for personal care, cleaning, and all our household requirements. We always joked, *"We don't have a medicine cabinet. We have a vitamin drawer in the kitchen."* Our health insurance was: *"Don't get sick. Just live as healthy and stress-free a life as possible."* We'd had health insurance for many years when we worked for other people, but with both of us self-employed, health insurance was just too costly to maintain.

Now our lives were about to change. After thousands of dollars in medical expenses so far, we raced to get my husband some excellent health insurance. But we would still need to make co-pays and cough up deductibles, which were expensive. And, my husband had his own small business as a computer consultant. How would we manage with him out of work? How could we keep his business going and weather all this? I knew we needed a game plan - fast! We needed lists, schedules, tools, and resources to stay on track. Everything was happening quickly. We needed to put the brakes on and think long and hard about what we were getting into, what we were giving up, and how to manage it all without going nuts.

After shedding a few tears, I rolled up my sleeves and decided to take control of the situation. We needed to buy some time to make a plan, rearrange our lives, get help running my husband's very active business, get health insurance, line up some help with basic things like who would walk and feed our dogs when we expected to be gone for these long treatment days. And who could help out occasionally with running errands, transportation to and from medical appointments, and housecleaning. And how we would manage financially. We asked our doctors if we could wait one month before beginning treatments and reluctantly, they agreed. But the clock was ticking and the pressure was on us to make the most of just a few precious weeks.

Before my husband was diagnosed with cancer, I had never taken care of anyone with a debilitating disease and it was a shock to suddenly be thrust into the role of fulltime caregiver. I've never been the "nursing type." I've always avoided dealing with *ooey-gooey* things. I could never imagine myself choosing to go through chemo and radiation, and I rarely go to "Western doctors." But this was his life and his choice and I decided to be supportive of whatever he needed to do to become whole, happy, and healthy again.

While I desperately needed a break, I knew it would have to wait. I had to jump in with both feet and deal with it all, whether I liked it or not, or whether I agreed with anything or not. I was highly skeptical of the whole process. I was angry, terrified, and in disbelief. But I found the strength I never knew I had to get through it all; to rally and be a cheerleader for my husband; to take things in stride; to focus, get things done, and just plain make things happen. All with a healthy dose of humor, too. And so can you.

So here's my advice to you from all that I learned:

Take charge of the situation you're in. Don't be swept along, dazed and confused. Be proactive - and do whatever you can to help your loved one heal and deal with things as best they can. Question the treatments and advice you are receiving until you understand what's happening. And, if something doesn't feel right in your gut, be sure to say, *"Is this necessary?" "Do we have to"*? Or *"What will happen if we don't?"* Then weigh your options before making a decision or adopting a point of view.

Toward the end of my husband's treatment when he was in the most pain, fear, and discomfort, one of the nurses told me, *"It will get much worse for him before he gets better. Your worst week is ahead of you."* This didn't feel right to me, as my husband had already been through what looked to me like the worst of it. I thought, *"Why does it have to be that way?"* So I asked her, *"Do we have to have that experience? Will it really have to be that way?"* I did not want to expect or imagine that things would get any worse. And guess what? I was not in denial, I was right! The worst was already over. We did not have the negative experience she described. So don't assume that everyone else's experience will be yours. Trust your instincts. This is where *"Mommy Medicine"* comes into play (*Chapter 15*). Listen to your heart and your gut. Pay attention. Observe your own situation and measure that against what you are being told. You probably know more than you think you do!

While the doctors did their best, we needed more information than they could provide. Their job was to give my husband the best protocols available to cure his cancer. But they were not prepared to help us organize our daily lives, and did not offer us checklists, shopping lists, and nutritional advice. Luckily, that is my area of expertise and why I wrote this book.

Introduction

While there is plenty of research to support the latest protocols, each patient is different. Symptoms vary widely. Doctors are uncertain which ones their patients will have, when they will happen, and how long they will last. And they don't want to frighten their patients and caregivers unnecessarily. While I didn't want to terrify myself by doing endless research on the web *(and I didn't)*, I still wanted to be prepared for whatever happened. And, while I wished the doctors could have provided more guidance on what to expect and when - perhaps I would not have been as proactive if I had been given *"a script."* This turned out to be a blessing in disguise.

Yes, the treatments were very difficult and painful. At one point my husband wanted to throw in the towel it was so bad. And, yes - it was a great strain on me at times, as well. But because we had made a plan, stayed flexible, and got lots of support from family and friends, we weathered the storm and came out the other side. A bit tattered, but certainly not destroyed. I just wish I'd had this book! So pour yourself a cup of tea, sit down, and read, dear ones. And know that help is on the way.

Chapter 3

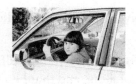

What This Book Is/Isn't Intended To Do...

This book IS NOT intended to:

- Diagnose an illness or replace medical advice from your doctors and health care practitioners.

- Prove that anyone or anything is right or wrong.

- Tell you what you should or shouldn't do.

- Offer advice to those who need surgery to remove their throat cancer tumor.

- Offer technical or scientific information. It does not inform you of the mechanics or causes of your cancer. Your doctor can provide you with facts, statistics, pictures, and studies that pertain to your cancer. There are also excellent websites for that purpose. You can find some of them listed in the resources section of this book.

- Deal with end of life decisions and issues facing terminal patients. For these concerns, consult your doctor and your local Hospice group.

This book IS intended to:

- Help with the "human side of cancer" - how it may affect your life, how to stay organized and sane, and how you can be as prepared and effective as possible at dealing with the healing and recovery process.

- Provide some comfort for you in these difficult times, letting you know that you are not alone and that help is available.

- Offer some advice from our personal experience to help simplify your life, get the help you need, and support the healing process as best you can.

- Give you some ideas and guidance on getting organized, shopping for supplies, nutritional needs, etc.

- Give you some resources for nutritional products, web sites to visit, etc.

- Help empower and encourage you to take charge of your medical situation by asking questions, doing whatever you can to make things work for you and your loved one, and making the choices and decisions that are right for you.

- Help you be resourceful and "think outside the box" when it comes to reorganizing your daily life.

- Encourage you to examine your medical bills and find solutions for paying them in full and on time.

- Help you understand that everyone is different and that you need to pay attention to your particular circumstance and what you need. Not everyone with throat cancer will experience the same symptoms, or even have the exact same treatments as my husband did. Your treatment regime will be tailored to your specific needs depending on how big the cancer is, where it is located, how long you've had it, and why you got it in the first place.

Chapter 4

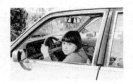

How To Use This Book

Use the whole book, just one chapter, or just one piece of advice. It is entirely up to you. Chapters are designed to address the various questions and concerns you may have right now.

If you read nothing else in this book, be sure to read the *General Advice* chapters for patients and caregivers *(Chapters 5 & 6)*. After that, read whatever chapters are most helpful to you right now. If you are at the beginning of the process, you don't have a lot of time. With that in mind, I did my best to keep things simple, straightforward, and to the point.

Before your loved one begins treatment, be sure to check out Chapter 21 for an idea of the kinds of tools, equipment and supplies you'll need to have on hand. Having an arsenal of kitchen gadgets and nutritional supplies will make your life easier.

To learn more about getting the best nutrition without using the standard, pre-packaged cans of liquid nutrition, be sure to read Chapter 18 - *Getting the Best Nutrition.* I've put together lots of useful information for you there.

If you need help with getting organized or looking at what parts of your life need to be rearranged right now, read Chapter 10 *(Staying Organized)* and Chapter 8 *(Make Plans Before Treatment Begins)*.

If you need to figure out how you're going to make it through the whole cancer ordeal financially, be sure to check out Chapter 11 *(no pun intended!) - Managing Your Mountain of Medical Bills*.

And if you're feeling stressed or emotionally charged, look at Chapters 22 and 23 for tips on staying sane, de-stressing, and finding the humor. Perspective is everything!

Chapter 5

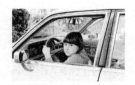

General Advice
for the Patient

Before treatment:
1. **Don't panic.** Throat cancer often shows up at "Stage 4," which means something entirely different than stage 4 in other cancers. It is one of the cancers that can actually be cured. You just might be one of the lucky ones, so get all the facts and ask lots of questions.
2. **Ask for help** for whatever you need. There is a lot of help available. Just ask!
3. **Take time to think things through** before you get started with chemo, radiation, etc. Don't be rushed to the medical altar. If you want a second or third opinion - or just want to meet other doctors before you select your team, by all means do. Having confidence in your medical team will make all the difference in the world to your healing process. Your clinic should be a "safe place to fall" - not a chaotic, fearful experience that causes you to feel greater anxiety.
4. **Get organized** and formulate a plan for how you're going to get through the next 3 critical months. Your life will be turned upside down for a while, but not forever. Your daily routine will change - as you'll need to make your treatments, nutrition, healing, and rest the biggest priority in your life. Ask your doctors if you can wait a week, two weeks, or a month before you start treatment. Unless you live an

extremely simple life with few responsibilities to others, you'll need time to get re-organized so your life will run as smoothly as possible.

5. **Line up your helpers.** In the American healthcare system, family members are expected to take care of the patients when they are at home. This means helping with cleaning wounds, changing bandages, and in some cases, helping you use your feeding tube for meals and hydration. You'll need help with all these things, plus grocery shopping, housecleaning, doing laundry and changing your bedding, walking and feeding pets, transportation to medical appointments, cooking, picking up medications for you, etc. If you live alone, have someone - or a few someones - take turns staying with you. If you spike a fever or have other health emergencies, you'll need a loved one or caregiver to watch over you and ask for help from your doctors.

6. **See a dentist before you begin treatments.** This may sound a bit crazy, but if you have the luxury of a few more weeks before the start of radiation for throat cancer, make sure you don't have any metal fillings or crowns in your mouth. If at all possible, have them replaced with ceramic or other non-metal fillings. One of my husband's most painful and debilitating symptoms was radiation burns in his mouth from radiation *"scatter,"* which is when radiation hits metal and bounces around. The scatter burns made it extremely difficult to eat - and even drinking water was painful. A relatively quick and effective method of replacing crowns is the *Cerec* process, a ceramic crown that is a same-day procedure. *Cerec* is an amazing breakthrough in technology that keeps improving and may really help you right now. It's worth checking into.

7. **Be prepared for a full range of emotional responses from others** when you tell them you have cancer. While some

people will be amazingly kind, generous, and sympathetic - others might be scared, angry, worried, distant, or even hostile. Hopefully, you'll get all the caring and support you need, but if not, don't take it personally. Conversations about cancer can consciously or unconsciously trigger people into dealing with their own mortality issues and many people are not prepared to handle this emotionally charged subject. It is not your fault. Just take a Zen approach when you can. Notice their reactions, but don't take them on.

During treatment:
1. **Keep things as simple as possible.** Try to create simple routines, e.g., if it's easiest for you to get most of your calories by making a great smoothie every day, do just that. Check out Chapter 20 for our favorite smoothie recipes that can give you the calories and nutrition you need using whole foods.
2. **Cut back on your work schedule.** So you're thinking, *"Can I work a normal schedule?"* It depends on what you do, how much and how often your treatments are, and whether or not you'll need a feeding tube. If you have primarily a desk job and work from home - and you don't need to talk to anyone by phone, you can expect to be able to work a reduced schedule. Otherwise, you'll need to take some time off. Why? Your voice may sound raspy, gravelly, or froggy; you will probably have dry mouth; you will probably feel a frequent urge to clear your throat, cough, and spit; you may be in a considerable amount of pain; you may be *"spacey"* from your medications and treatments; you might have a fever off and on; and if you have a feeding tube, you'll have this crazy thing sticking out of your stomach that will protrude through your clothes and might leak. You may feel

downright cranky and irritable - a lot! If you've got a public job in a public place, are you prepared to feed yourself through your feeding tube? Do you have privacy and access to a personal bathroom? Are you being fair to your co-workers, etc., by imposing your illness, mood swings, and needs on them? Please think this through.

3. **Get help with transportation** to and from your oncologists and other doctors. While you might be able to drive to and from your treatments and other medical visits, it's not a great idea. Here's why: you may be tired, in pain, distracted, easily upset, angry, or just plain *"loopy"* from the various medications you'll be prescribed. Some of the drugs you may be given will act as if you are *"under the influence."* In fact, if you're pulled over for a driving infraction while on these medications, you'll be treated as if you are DUI. In the long run, having someone drive you to and from your treatments will be a great relief. It's one less thing you need to worry about.

4. **Always bring an advocate to your doctor appointments.** You could experience a feeling of being *"foggy"* - and your memory might not be as sharp as it usually is. You may be in pain, which can cloud your thinking. You may also be *"foggy"* from just being on overload from all that is happening to you. This is why bringing your spouse or a trusted friend, family member, or caregiver to your doctor visits is a great idea. Have them sit in on your checkups and evaluations. This is no time to be shy. Your advocate can provide more objectivity than you. They will be able to hear what the doctor is telling you and take appropriate notes, etc. It may be hard for you to focus, and words may *"go in one ear and out the other"* for a while. Let your advocate provide stability for you and allow them to be your eyes and ears at the doctor's office. Your health advocate can also be invaluable at giving

your doctors feedback about your condition, needs, concerns, changing symptoms, etc.

5. **Stock up on supplies you'll need.** Try to have enough food, medical supplies, etc., on hand so that you or your caregiver doesn't have to shop every day. (*See Chapter 21 on what you'll need to have on hand.*)

6. **Have your feeding tube operation early in the process.** If your doctor recommends getting a feeding tube, get it done earlier rather than later in the treatment process. Early on, you'll undoubtedly have more strength and stamina, so ask your doctor to schedule your feeding tube procedure within the first ten days of treatment or so. Yes, it hurts. Yes, there is some downtime and recovery time from this procedure. And, there is some adjustment time to having a feeding tube in your tummy. You'll need to learn how to use it, how to clean it, and how to deal with it emotionally as well as physically. Give yourself the time you need to make it as easy and convenient as possible. And go easy on yourself. This is unlike anything you've ever experienced before - and hopefully, will never have to experience again.

7. **Eat healthy, real food by mouth for as long as possible.** Keeping your throat muscles active and working will help with the recovery process. If solids are too painful to swallow - drink liquids, smoothies, and pureed foods. Find what works for you. (*See Chapter 18 on nutrition.*)

8. **Do whatever it takes to keep your spirits up.** Watch funny movies, read inspirational stories, get a joke book. Take walks in beautiful places. Meditate. (*See Chapter 22 on Staying Sane for more tips.*)

9. **Keep things as normal as possible.** If you're used to being out and about and seeing people, then do just that. Don't isolate yourself unless you enjoy isolation. Meet a friend for coffee (*Yes - you can drink coffee - just not too hot or too cold.*) Try

something soft and easy to eat on the menu like scrambled
eggs, pancakes with syrup, or creamy soups.

10. **Get the rest you need.** Treatments can be exhausting both
    physically and emotionally. Go home and rest afterwards.
    And when treatments are complete, you'll need rest for
    several more weeks. Reintegrate back into your life slowly
    and give yourself a break, if possible. You're more likely to
    recover more quickly if you take time to rest and recuperate
    when your body needs it the most. This is not a *"pedal to the
    metal"* time in your life.

11. **Remember to say thank you** and express your appreciation
    to those who are helping you, including your medical team.
    If family and friends are helping out, what matters most is
    not how much or how often they give to you, but how much
    they care and support you during this tumultuous time.

After treatment:

1. **Take it slow.** Don't expect to *"hit the ground running"* once
   treatments are over. Recovery takes time and you've still got
   a lot of healing to do. Go easy on yourself and get all the
   extra rest and recuperation you need.

2. **Continue asking for help.** Daily chores can still be
   exhausting, so be sure to ask for help whenever you need it.
   No one will expect you to be back to normal yet.

3. **Be patient.** Symptoms will continue for awhile, so be
   prepared to pay extra attention to your body's needs, such as
   additional care of the radiated skin, etc.

4. **Slowly integrate eating by mouth.** If you have mouth sores,
   they may continue for several more weeks to come, but they
   will subside. Start eating *"real meals"* when you feel up to it -
   but keep the food soft and easy to eat and digest. No salsa!

5. **Keep up the extra calories.** It may take many more months
   before you can eat a normal amount of calories. Just enjoy

the extra goodies while everyone else is jealous of the desserts you can eat!

6. **Consider a part-time schedule** when resuming work or your normal life until you regain your strength. Easy does it.

7. **Have the feeding tube removed** once you're back to eating all your meals by mouth. The removal process is a simple, outpatient procedure that should be pretty straightforward and painless. You can expect to have it removed 4-6 weeks after treatments end.

8. **Check with your doctor** for any questions or concerns you may have, for any symptoms you don't understand, and to learn more about what to expect in the way of healing. You'll continue to have regular medical follow-ups and tests, further and further apart. Typical follow-ups are at one month, three months, then every six months depending on test results. Follow-up PET scans are usually one year after treatment ends.

9. **Visualize yourself being cancer-free and enjoying life.** Start noticing the progress you're making. Small improvements will add up over time. Start reintegrating into your life the things you love doing.

10. **Think positive!** You're in the home stretch!

Chapter 6

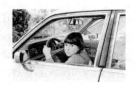

General Advice
for the Caregiver

1. **Don't panic.** This book should help you understand what's going on and what steps you can take to get organized and see things through as effectively as possible.
2. **Get educated.** Read Chapter 14 on *Symptoms and Side Effects*, Chapter 12 on the *Feeding Tube*, and learn what tools and supplies you'll need in Chapter 21. And if you're inclined to create excellent nutrition for the patient, be sure to read Chapter 18.
3. **Get organized.** Read Chapter 10. It's designed to make your life easier.
4. **Ask for help.** Whether you are a spouse, partner, family member, or friend, get support. Do what you do best, and if at all possible, delegate the rest. Share the cooking and errands. Get help with driving the patient to their appointments. Have someone else walk the dogs and give you a break from washing dishes. You might be able to *do it all*, but this is not a great plan. You'll get burnout, get cranky and resentful, and you won't be as effective in the long run if you don't get some relief.
5. **Remember to take good care of yourself.** You need nurturing, too. Don't skip meals. My recipe chapter has meals designed to feed both you and the patient (*Chapter 20*).

6. **Do whatever it takes to stay centered.** Read Chapters 22 and 23 on *Staying Sane* and *Seeing the Humor.*

7. **Bring some happiness with you to the waiting rooms.** The waiting rooms can zap your energy with all the pain and sadness there. Patients and their caregivers are often frightened, in pain, or very sad. Refrain from *"tuning in"* to the pain around you and do what you can to stay centered. For instance, I got permission to bring my two perky little dogs (*fluffy little Bichons*) to the radiation clinic. They not only cheered me up, they enjoyed meeting everyone there and brought happiness to many people. Our waiting room changed almost overnight from a quiet place where people wiped away their tears - to a congenial group that looked forward to seeing the dogs and us every day. Think outside the box. What can you do to bring more joy into the world?

8. **Use this experience as an opportunity for growth.** This may very well be the perfect opportunity for you to find your strength, take charge, take on a new challenge, or learn something new. Or, all of the above!

9. **Use this experience as an opportunity to practice being more loving,** kind, and compassionate. Keep a good sense of humor whenever you can. Look for the silver lining in whatever experiences come your way. Stay positive!

10. **Be a cheerleader for your loved one.** Muster up the energy, strength, joy, happiness, and positive outlook to cheer them on. The patient will most likely not have the capacity or reserves to stay in a positive mindset. They may be in various stages of pain, grief, etc. It may be up to you to provide stability to their daily life and to cheer them on during this grueling time.

11. **Be supportive as much and as often as you can.** Your loved one needs to count on you and lean on you at a time in their life when they may be very scared and unable to gain

perspective. You are there to provide the loving support they need now more than ever.

12. **Be grateful for what you have** and remember to find the beauty and joy in the little miracles in daily life. Small gestures of kindness and caring can mean more than you realize right now - from you toward others and from others toward you.

A special note about caregivers in America:

As I write this, one of the great tragedies in the American medical and health insurance system is that the system expects and forces the patient's family members to do the work that nurses used to do - whether or not family members or friends possess the knowledge, skills, experience, or emotional and psychological stamina to do so. In addition, a request for a nurse to help the patient at home is considered a rather unnecessary and in some cases laughable request. The patient's spouse and/or family are just supposed to roll up their sleeves and do whatever it takes. While this started as both a cost savings method for the insurance companies and on a positive note - an opportunity for families to care for their loved ones at home, the system has broken down to the point that family members are given no choice about caretaking. It's their job. Period. End of story. Question this rule if you feel so inclined. I certainly did. Most health insurance policies will only cover a nurse coming to the patient's home *to train* a spouse or family member on caretaking, not to actually provide home health care services. This is yet one more burdensome responsibility the American family has been forced to bear. Hopefully, that will change for the better in the not-too-distant future.

That being said, I asked for and received help from the wonderful nursing staffs at both the chemo and the radiation centers in terms of feeding my husband by feeding tube and changing his bandages. I was pretty worn out by the end of my husband's cancer treatments, and I especially needed extra help at that time. This was definitely a case of *"ask and you shall receive."* Everyone was very helpful and compassionate toward us and we were grateful and appreciative for their support. It's o.k. to ask for help. Preserve yourself, *please.*

Chapter 7

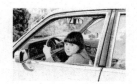

What This Is and Isn't The Right Time to *Do-Be-Do-Be-Do*

This is not the right time to ...

1. Resolve all your unresolved conflicts and emotional problems.
2. Take care of other people.
3. Do everything yourself.
4. Ask for help from people who cannot give this to you. This includes people who are either emotionally, physically, or financially incapable of being there for you.
5. Focus on your regrets.
6. Blame yourself or be judgmental toward yourself or others.
7. Behave badly or take your anger and frustrations out on those who love you, care about you, or care for you.
8. Waste time defending your decisions and choices to family and friends - especially those who tend to be difficult or judgmental.
9. Ask yourself, *"Why me?"* or have a pity party.
10. Allow yourself to get depressed.
11. Worry and freak out.
12. Allow yourself to be bullied or forced into doing things you don't agree with or understand.
13. Push people away who are sincerely trying to help you.
14. Indulge in negative thinking.

15. Throw tantrums.
16. Decide to not show up for your medical appointments and treatments.
17. Act self-destructively by not taking good care of yourself.
18. Throw in the towel and give up.

This is the right time to ...
1. Connect with people who love and support you.
2. Allow in people who are kind and eliminate the bozos.
3. Set strong boundaries.
4. Focus on your healing and wellness and getting through the process.
5. Ask for help.
6. Look for the blessings in your life. Even noticing small, special things can make a big difference in your outlook on life.
7. Rest whenever you need to.
8. Say "thank you" and be appreciative to those who are helping you.
9. Focus on what you **can** do, not on what you can't.
10. Watch your mood swings and do your best to keep your emotions in check.
11. Muster up the courage to see things through.
12. Notice your negative feelings and write about them if it helps - and - avoid getting stuck in them, if at all possible. A lot of what is happening to you is temporary. Symptoms, experiences, pain, etc., may come and go and will most definitely change.
13. Know that you will not be like this forever. You will not be suffering and in pain forever. You will get better.
14. Picture yourself improving every day. Picture the cancer cells diminishing until they are all gone.

15. Speak up when you need more information about your medical condition and/or treatment. Speak up if the medical system, billing system, insurance system, or health care providers need to be paying more attention to something that is not right or that needs to be changed. Know that you are helping them improve which will result in helping others in your situation, as well.

16. Write some affirmations for yourself and read them every day. Here is one of my favorites: *"Each day is a blessing filled with love, kindness, caring, inspiration, joy, strength, vitality, ease, laughter, good fortune, and heartwarming miracles."*

17. Have faith. Trust. Look forward to a brighter future. If life throws you curve balls down the road, deal with it then. Worrying about what may or may not happen isn't going to help you feel any better right now.

18. Ask questions and get the answers you need so you can have greater understanding, awareness, and peace of mind.

19. Be proactive about your health. Take charge of your situation.

20. Close your eyes and visualize a *"stop sign"* or say the word *"stop!"* whenever your negative thoughts and emotions take hold of you. Know that you can retrain your brain!

21. To the best of your ability, do things that are enjoyable to you and make you happy. Happiness, joy, and laughter are good for healing your body, mind, and soul.

22. Tell yourself, *"This too shall pass."*

23. See if you can find any humor in your situation. After all, this may very well be the craziest thing that's every happened to you. If it's not, you might consider doing stand-up comedy!

Chapter 8

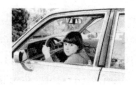

Make Plans
Before Treatment Begins

Before treatment begins, try to make plans for how you will manage your daily life and current responsibilities throughout the treatment process and beyond. Things will go much smoother for you if you plan ahead. As I mentioned in the General Advice chapter, please take a little time to get re-organized and it will make a world of difference. Here are some areas of your life that may need some extra planning:

Make a plan for how you will get through the next 2-3 months (*i.e., cancer treatment and the 4-6 weeks following treatment*). If you are working, realistically you'll need to reduce, share, or delegate your workload altogether so you can heal properly. The treatments are very intense and quite consuming. My husband's protocol included radiation treatments five days per week for 6-7 weeks. Chemo was administered once a week for the same amount of weeks. You could probably handle working more if the treatment regime was once every 3-6 weeks, but an everyday regime can be exhausting. In our case, my husband started out being able to work and actually brought his laptop to chemo. But that process quickly changed, especially after the pain kicked in. He was not thinking clearly or making good decisions - and he knew it. If your job requires management, problem-solving, quick decision-making, physical stamina, heavy lifting, public appearances, or in-person communications with clients or staff, you'll definitely need some time off and will probably need to fully or partially delegate responsibilities to someone else while you recuperate.

Please consider these work-related issues before treatment begins:

- Can you survive financially without a steady paycheck for 3 months or more?

- Can you work from home at all?

- Can you take a leave of absence or only work part time?

- Whether you have an employer or own your own business, is there anyone available who can share your workload and responsibilities?

- If you own a business, can you rearrange or reduce your work schedule to accommodate your health needs?

- If you're a sole proprietor or small business owner, are you the only one who can do your work or make major decisions? Or, is there someone who can help run the business for you while you're gone?

My husband has a small business and we had to find ways to keep it up and running not only while my husband was undergoing chemo and radiation, but for an additional month after treatments, as well. As a sole proprietor, he was used to running everything himself and not asking for help. I had to jump in with both feet and become much more of a partner in his business, which I still am to this day. I hired other people to take his place, helped keep the business running, dealt with his customers to keep the business flourishing, and brought work home for my husband to do at his own pace when he felt up to it. This was no small feat! If I was not in the picture or did not get help from my husband's colleagues, I don't think his business would have survived his absence.

If you don't have to work or can find a way to take time off, you'll be much better off, especially when you're in the thick of treatments. In the U.S. we often make work the most important thing. It's not. You are! We're also taught to *"tough it out"* and not ask for help. This is definitely not the time to be a lone cowboy. Ask for help!

Plan how you will manage financially and how you will pay your bills:
See the chapter entitled: Managing your Mountain of Medical Bills

Plan how you will manage your daily life:
The patient will undoubtedly need more rest during the day and more sleep at night. They will experience more exhaustion than they are normally used to. Simple, everyday tasks such as cooking, cleaning, running errands, etc., can be quite challenging for someone undergoing throat cancer treatments. If a feeding tube is installed, it can be difficult for the patient to comfortably bend and lift and they will probably be weak from all the weight loss. Simple activities such as changing bedding and doing laundry can be challenging and frustrating. Help will be needed.

If you are alone, consider having a friend or relative come and help out. This is a tough protocol to do alone. If you need to administer salves and soaks at home for the neck area, some treatments are more effective if done while the patient is lying down. This is very difficult to do on yourself. You will need help with this. If a friend or relative can't help out *(or even if they can)*, consider asking your doctor for a prescription for a home health aid or nurse.

Plan for extra help at home:
Caregiving during this time can be a fulltime job. Whether you're the caregiver or the patient, you'll need all the help you can get. Even if you have a spouse or partner who can help take care of you, they will undoubtedly need a break from time to time. I was overwhelmed and exhausted from all the constant caretaking, errands, food prep, and driving to and from medical appointments. Fortunately, a few gracious siblings stayed for extended periods of time to help us out, which was great. It was also wonderful for me to have support and camaraderie during such a difficult time. In addition, some of our friends helped run errands, cared for our pets on chemo days, and pitched in to do some of the driving to and from John's medical appointments. This was a godsend.

Plan for your chemo days:
My husband's chemo treatments took 4-6 hours to administer and were followed by radiation. These were our toughest days by far, as his long absences from work and home forced us to plan ahead. The patient will need to bring their special food *(canned or otherwise)*, any medicines they are taking, supplies for various symptoms *(e.g., Biotene gum for dry mouth)*, a change of clothes, work and/or reading materials, a laptop, cell phone, etc. See my suggestions for a *"To Go"* kit further on in this chapter.

If you have pets, you may need to arrange help for their walking and feeding. If school-aged children are at home, you'll need to arrange for pickups and drop-offs from school or other activities, as well as meals, caretaking, etc.

Additionally, you'll need help with transportation to and from chemo, as it can be physically and emotionally draining - not only from the treatment itself, but also from spending the better part of a day surrounded by people who are suffering. My husband usually slept or rested on the way home from chemo. He was not at all *"up for driving"* and was very grateful to have me there to help.

After chemo, patients can have a variety of symptoms, including fevers, nausea, allergic reactions, exhaustion, or just not feeling well in general. You may need additional help at home. If you live alone, arrange for someone to either stay with you that night or check in on you before bedtime to make sure you're o.k.

Plan a "To-Go" kit:
Because we were on the road so much due to my husband's medical appointments and related errands, we always packed a "To-Go Kit."Our kit changed as his symptoms and needs changed, but because of his eating, medication, and personal care routines, we needed to bring things with us. Consider bringing whatever you need to take care of yourself if you plan on being on the road for a couple of hours or more. Your to-go kit should include bottles of water and/or juice, food, medicines, salves and ointments for the radiated skin, etc. In addition, we brought a bottle of nasal saline, cough drops, Biotene gum, bandages and tape, disposable gloves, travel-

sized applesauce, and extra bandanas. Don't assume your doctors will have all the tools and supplies you need. Just bring whatever you need. For a complete list, see our checklist chapter.

Plan for how/where you will take care of yourself when you're in the outside world:

When you're away from home, you'll need access to clean, private bathrooms where you can take care of your personal care regimes. These may include changing bandages, feeding by feeding tube, and cleaning the feeding tube. These can be messy activities as well as procedures that can make you vulnerable to infection. Some of these caretaking processes can be bloody, disturbing, and downright gross. Unless you're doing a supervised demonstration for medical students, your personal care regimes should be done privately. So be sure to make a plan for where you can take care of yourself away from the public eye.

Plan something to look forward to:

Most importantly, make plans to incorporate something fun or enjoyable into your daily or weekly regime. Whether you prefer to stay home and watch movies or have the energy to go out, be sure to add in some activities that make you happy. Skydiving and scuba diving will need to wait, and you probably won't feel much like partying. But, you can certainly visit with friends, take walks in a beautiful place, go out for coffee, go to the movies, and more. Just try.

Chapter 9

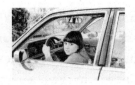

Asking For Help

Most people have a difficult time asking for help, but understand that you'll need extra support right now. If you're the type of person who either feels uncomfortable imposing on other people or is more comfortable giving than receiving, you now have an opportunity to try something new. Don't go it alone if you don't have to. People are more understanding than you think. Ask for help. Hopefully, your most high-intensity throat cancer demands will be very short-lived (*3 months*).

For the patient, it's not easy to give up control, but in some instances it's the best course of action - especially for safety reasons (*e.g., driving a car*). Some medicines may mask how impaired the patient really is. I often used to kid with my husband when we were heading to his treatment appointments saying, *"I'll drive. You're not that o.k."* And we'd laugh.

If you enjoy mobilizing support through online communities, I recently learned about a website that does just that: www.LotsaHelpingHands.com. The site is designed to help you ask for help by listing what needs to get done (*shopping, driving, housecleaning, etc.*) and putting the word out to family and friends so they can sign up for specific tasks. This can be a great tool for getting the help you need in an unobtrusive way. While it is a less personal approach, it may be easier for you to ask for help in this way. Just remember that there are still some people out there who would prefer a more personal approach when being asked for help.

If family and friends are far-flung and you don't have support nearby from people you love and trust, you have a couple of options. Ask your clinic or health insurance for a list of licensed and approved home health aids in your area. Also, there are volunteers available through a variety of groups and organizations, including: local cancer support organizations, church groups, and even your clinic. In our area, for example, we have a church-related volunteer group that helps patients with their transportation needs to and from doctor appointments.

For other types of support with daily life, in some cities there are wonderful services for delivering groceries and running other errands. Many dry cleaners also offer laundry services and some of them will pick up and deliver, as well. There are housekeeping services, personal chefs, and personal shoppers. For pet owners, there are dog walkers, pet sitters, and doggie daycare facilities. There are also mobile vet services and mobile grooming services that will come to your home or office, as well. Ask your vet for their list of recommended vendors for any pet-related services in your area.

This is a time to "call in the troops," so don't be shy about asking for help. After all, if not now, when? Leaning on others for support right now can be exactly what the doctor ordered, so to speak. And if you need to call on "the kindness of strangers" through a church group or cancer volunteer group, just do it. They're happy to help!

Chapter 10

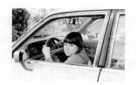

Staying Organized
and Keeping it Simple

How do you stay ahead of the game when everything keeps changing? The trick is to get organized, simplify and streamline routines, and stay as flexible and good-humored as you can. I've found the more organized I am, the better equipped I am to handle whatever challenges and changes are thrown my way. And this puts me in a good mood!

So relax, take a breath, and let me give you a few suggestions for making life just a little bit easier during this crazy and uncertain time.

Rule #1: Find a way to streamline things. If you hit on something that works, make it part of your daily routine.

Rule #2: Stay as organized as you possibly can. Keep a treatment notebook and write down the things you'll need to remember. Make lists of whatever you need. In the long run, staying organized will reduce your stress.

Rule #3: Find ways to let people help. Don't go it alone or you'll burn out. Besides, people who love and care about you will want to help in whatever way they can.

Rule #4: Simplify whatever needs to be done. If adding new regimes makes your life more difficult or more complicated, try to find solutions that will make your life easier. You don't need any more stress right now.

Rule #5: Add shifts and changes gradually. Don't try to change everything all at once. For example, if the patient needs to make dietary or lifestyle changes, make them in increments. Add changes slowly. If you've been eating a typical American diet, start shifting your pattern by adding more fresh veggies. Remove favorite *(but unhealthy)* foods gradually.

Rule #6: Go easy on yourself. This really is a challenging time.

Tips for staying organized
There's no great mystery for getting organized. Just write everything down. Don't even try to remember everything right now. It's just not possible. Make lists. Lists can help you streamline your errands, stay on track with medications, help you remember the patient's ever-changing symptoms, and help anyone who is assisting you.

Keep track of things on something portable
Whether it's a mobile device, a computer, or a pad of yellow paper and pen in a notebook, it doesn't matter. What matters is that you keep track in a way that works for you and will help you remember what needs to get done and when. Never underestimate the value of a yellow sticky!

Keep a "To Do" list

"To Do Lists" are great. You don't have to remember all the errands you need to run or the things you need to take care of. Consider this your cheat sheet on everything that needs to get done and when. I usually divide mine into the following: Calls to make, Emails to send and Internet *"to do's"* (*e.g., websites to visit, etc.*), Correspondence, Errands to run, Bills to pay, Miscellaneous, and Notes. Again - whether you write these on a pad of paper, in your calendar, or on an electronic device really doesn't matter. Just choose the right method for you to stay on track.

Make a list of your contacts and resources

Make a caregiver's list - of all the doctors, clinics, and pharmacies, involved with the patient's care - along with their addresses, phone numbers, email addresses, etc. Your resource list should include a list of the patient's family member's phone numbers and emergency contacts, as well. If the patient has school age children, make sure their school info and doctors are on the list. Also, if the patient has any pets, be sure to include their vet on this list.

Make a copy of your resource list to leave at home or set it up so you can email it. Perhaps you are the type who keeps all your info on a mobile device. That's great. Just be sure if anyone else is taking care of the patient, etc. - they will have easy access to this information as well - especially if an emergency arises.

Make a checklist for medicines and home care routines

Make a list of any medicines the patient needs to take and how often. When my husband was on some serious pain medication, we kept a checklist of dates and times for taking medicine on a yellow, lined pad of paper on the counter near his medicine. It made things easier. No one needed to remember if medicine had been taken or not. We just wrote it all down. We did this with several of his medicines. Alternatively, you can set your mobile device, computer, or wristwatch alarm to remind you when to administer medicine, if that's easier and more convenient for you.

Make a list for the doctor(s)

Keep a list of symptoms the patient is experiencing as well as questions you and the patient have. Be sure to bring these with you to the doctor's office. There's a good chance either you or the patient will draw a blank under duress, as being at an oncology clinic can be quite stressful as well as intimidating or upsetting.

Additionally, bring something to take notes on while at the doctor's office. And, have a folder or notebook for handouts. You'll be given instructions on what you'll need to buy, bring, or do - and you'll need to write these down. Don't assume you'll be provided with the information or checklists you'll need, as every patient is different.

Create a food/calorie log

Keep a food diary to track what the patient eats and how many calories they consume. This is essential, especially if you're not using pre-measured, canned nutrition. We kept a food diary as well as a daily time log of when my husband needed to achieve certain calorie goals. This helped him tremendously by helping him work at getting most of his calories by mid-afternoon. As a result, he did not have to push to eat a lot more at the end of the day, when he was more exhausted and just wanted to rest.

Simplify treatment schedules

If at all possible, try to schedule the cancer treatments for the same time each day or week. It will be much easier to remember and you will create more stability in your daily routines when you're not switching from one time slot to another.

Allow extra time for daily routines

Make sure you allow more time to get ready in the morning, around mealtimes, at bedtime, and in your bathing routines. There will be extra food prep, feeding, bathing, and personal care requirements. And, extra time will be needed before and after meals for cleaning the feeding tube. There will be medicines to take and keep track of and possibly bandages to change. When planning your day, be sure to factor in extra time to accommodate these new regimes so you don't get frustrated or run late.

Streamline errands and shopping

Whether you're the one who's shopping or not, it takes the stress out to not have to remember everything. Keep a running shopping list of whatever you need from the grocery stores, pharmacies, etc. This will maximize your efforts and cut down on time spent in stores.

Group items on your shopping list by category

For example: produce, personal care, dairy, frozen, etc. It's faster to shop that way, and if you can't find some of your items at one store, you'll easily know what types of things you'll need to find elsewhere if you keep a list by category, checking off what you already bought.

Organize prescriptions and medical supplies needed

If the doctor gives us prescriptions or suggests we purchase certain supplies, I keep their prescriptions and medical shopping list in my notebook. Then, when I'm out shopping, I have everything together in one place.

Tips to streamline cooking and prep

Have all your ingredients prepped, chopped, and ready to go before you start cooking. I find this much more efficient than prepping as I go. Often, I'll clean and chop a variety of vegetables when I have the chance in the morning. Or while I'm making a meal, I often just cut up extras of whatever ingredients I'm using - and put them in small bags in my fridge. Then they're ready to go when I need to cook. This cuts down on my cooking and prep time.

Buy pre-cut veggies and fruit when you can. There are lots of choices available. Just open the bag and you're good to go. Pre-washed, pre-cut fruits and veggies are great for making smoothies and soups. They cost a bit more, but what you need right now is time and simplicity. These puppies will do the trick!

Make double the recipe and freeze for later, such as meatloaves, soups, and even desserts. Meatloaves can be cut into individual servings and frozen. So can many soups and even desserts such as brownies. Just defrost and reheat, as needed. Easy peasy!

Other organizing essentials

Calendar

Keep a portable calendar for medical appointments. You can also write down and keep track of symptoms by date and time, as well.

This will come in handy for reporting any changes in symptoms to your oncology team.

Wills and Medical Power of Attorney
Make sure the patient has their will in order and up to date. Also - make sure they've filled out the form for a Medical Power of Attorney - the person who will be responsible for making important medical decisions should the patient be unable to do so themselves. This is especially important if the patient will be having surgery and will be unconscious during the procedure.

Keeping friends and family informed
Set up a page on *"Caring Bridge"* (*www.CaringBridge.org*) or something similar. Caring Bridge is a site designed to keep loved ones updated and informed about the patient's health condition. This is personal, private information and your privacy is respected. Signing up with a site like Caring Bridge saves you many precious hours that would otherwise be spent staying in touch with everyone individually. It's also a less stressful way of communicating than having to talk to everyone. The *Caring Bridge* web site proved to be a godsend for us. My husband enjoyed sitting down and writing essentially a blog for those he personally invited. It was great for him to receive well wishes on his site and great for his family and friends to keep up with his progress.

A note about simplifying
At this crazy time on planet earth, it can be a real challenge to simplify your life. In my country (*the U.S.*), the majority of Americans are working harder, putting in longer hours, and achieving less than

they had in the recent past. Welcome to the 21st century where the pace of life feels sped up, the future seems uncertain, and we're dancing as fast as we can just to keep up. As changes happen at breakneck speed, we're forced to constantly rearrange and readjust our lives. This can be exhausting! For most of us, adding cancer to the mix can throw our lives out of balance, making life completely unmanageable and overwhelming. Staying organized, streamlining, and simplifying your life wherever possible is the key to making it through this crazy cancer process. So do whatever it takes to make things easy on yourself.

Chapter 11

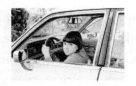

Managing Your Mountain of Medical Bills

Whether you have fabulous insurance, mediocre insurance, or no insurance at all, here are some tips to dealing with your medical bills. If paying medical bills is not an issue or a problem for you *(lucky you!)*, just skip this chapter. Or, if you're curious, read on ...

Rule #1: Don't assume the bills and invoices being sent to you are correct. In my experience, billing departments - whether in-house or outsourced - often send out bills that are either incorrect or not current. There are a whole host of reasons for this. Medical bills can reflect services the patient received several months ago - and even longer - and these services may have already been paid or partially paid by you or your insurance company. Sometimes, a billing department sends your bills to the wrong insurance company and it may take several tries to correct the problem. Also, billing departments may switch computer systems, computer programs, locations, or billing subcontractors. Bottom line: bills are usually computerized, computers were invented by humans, and humans are flawed. Computers and people make mistakes all the time. So, always make sure you have the most current and accurate medical bills before paying them.

If you can't pay your medical bills in full, don't panic. Most health care providers will work with you to create a payment plan if you need one. Some clinics and hospitals are more generous or lenient than others. Most do not charge interest. And, they are usually quite happy that you want to pay your bill and that you are in communication with them. Remember to write down who you spoke to and when - along with what was said during your conversation. Emailing is fine, but sometimes it's just more expedient to call instead of waiting for a response. And, always ask for the updated bills and payment arrangements to be mailed or emailed to you. You always want to have your agreements in writing.

Ask if you qualify to receive financial help. If you need help paying your bills, most facilities have someone on staff whose job it is to be knowledgeable about agencies that provide funding for your circumstance. Don't be afraid to ask for this information. There are local and national nonprofits that are set up to help. And, the clinics and hospitals may have funding, too. It's not unusual for donors to give money to specific cancer-related funds at these facilities. Just ask.

If you're unhappy, speak up! If you're sincerely unhappy with the service provided or the company you're doing business with, ask to speak to a supervisor. If you are dealing with a hospital, most facilities have an *Ombudsman* or *Patient Advocate* on staff. It's their job to check into complaints and see what they can do to fix the problems. They are there to listen to you and they want you to be a happy customer. Example: My husband and I were particularly upset with the way we were treated at the hospital where he had surgery.

After telling our story and complaining to the Ombudsman, they came back to us with a $1,000 reduction on our bill as an *"I'm sorry mistakes were made."* They later gave us 30% off of our bill, which amounted to several thousand dollars. It may very well pay to speak up and air your grievances!

Remember to negotiate. No one tells you that most medical bills are negotiable. It was a shock to us to learn this. Even the various insurance companies negotiate different rates with the same facility. When did our medical system turn into a flea market? Well - that's a subject for another book. If you get an outlandish medical bill, call the facility and ask, *"If I pay my bill in full now, what kind of discount can you give me?"* You can also ask if they can give you the Medicare rate - or the medical insurance company rate. We discovered that typical discounts for paying in full - either by check or credit card - range from 10% to 35%. That can be quite a substantial savings!

Question your medical bills - especially if you don't understand them. I can't tell you how many times I would call a billing department to ask about specific charges on a bill I had in front of me and they would end up saying, *"Disregard that charge. You don't owe anything."* I'm not kidding! Sometimes the charges were dropped because the health insurance already paid them. And in one instance, my husband noticed that our health insurance had paid the negotiated rate in full and the hospital was trying to get us to pay more than the negotiated rate. When we questioned why we should pay more, we got an email saying, *"It's no one's responsibility to pay the additional amount. Just disregard it. We took it off your bill."* We saved about $3,000.00 questioning our bills and finding out we didn't owe the billing amounts that were sent us. When in doubt, it's definitely worth making the calls.

Question any unusual fees and add a dash of humor. We noticed that some of our service providers were coming up with creative ways of making more money by adding unusual or unexpected fees. It's o.k. to question the validity of these fees and see if you can have them waived or reduced. Here's an example: About 4 months after my husband had a couple of follow-up visits with one of his doctors, we were billed almost $200 with a memo that said it was "past due." We had no idea what this bill referred to, since the doctor's bills and our co-payments had already been paid in full for those visits. The bill referenced the office visit dates with no further explanation. We called our health insurance company and they said the fees were for "Facilities Charges" and while they would apply them to our annual deductible, they would not pay them. What is a "Facilities Charge?" Good question. The clinic broke the bill into two parts: the fee for the doctor's services (*which our insurance gladly paid*) and then - tah dah - the fee for "using the facility," i.e., sitting in the waiting room, sitting in the doctor's office, going to the restroom, etc. I'm not kidding! The up-side of this experience is that it did provide us with hours of comedy ideas for lowering this fee, including: standing at the doctor's office instead of sitting (*standing on one leg might be even cheaper*); bringing our own toilet paper; and of course, bringing our own bucket to pee in. And, we were wondering how to break all the expenses down: using the scale: $15; reading a magazine in the waiting room: $20; etc. You get my point. So if you see fees that seem unfair or just plain ridiculous, question them. After all, where do we draw the line? Will we start being charged not just for our groceries, but also for standing in line at the grocery store? Or, if we try on clothes at a department store, will we have to pay for the items we buy as well as the time spent in the dressing room? I could go on and on about the ridiculousness of this fee. Bottom line: if you see a "Facilities Fee" for an outpatient clinic that is not located at a hospital, question this one. In my opinion, a facilities charge should be the clinic's cost of doing business, not your responsibility as a patient or caregiver to pay.

Pay by credit card if you really need to. I don't recommend paying medical bills with credit cards, but in a pinch, by all means do. Most clinics and hospitals take credit cards - even by phone. The main reason I don't want you to use credit cards is for the extra interest you'll be paying. Since clinics and hospitals don't usually charge interest or additional fees if you create a payment plan with them, why pay additional fees?

Ask for help from family and friends. But don't guilt-trip them into helping you. If you're lucky enough to have friends or family who are willing to help you financially, consider yourself very lucky - and remember to thank them!

Start a medical fund. Think big and think outside the box. When faced with the possibility that my husband's cancer-related medical bills could bankrupt us, we decided to open a new bank account to help pay off his bills and let friends and family contribute to it. Believe it or not, it is very easy to do. Just ask your bank what they need from you in order to create one. For us it was as simple as creating a name for an additional personal account and signing new signature cards. Our medical account was up and running in a couple of days, checks and all. If people want to be anonymous, let them know they can give financial gifts anonymously by just sending their checks directly to your medical fund bank account at a specific branch and asking to remain anonymous. You can arrange this with the branch manager. In our case, a number of people made contributions anonymously - and that was great.

Offer your friends and family ways to come through for you and they probably will if they can. In the case of my husband's medical fund - which he named the *Cancer Recovery Fund* - friends, family members, and clients were asking him, *"How can I help?"* Creating a medical fund proved to be a wonderful solution, and as a result, we did not have to consider bankruptcy as an option. We let people know that no gift was too small and all gifts would be appreciated. Because of the *Cancer Recovery Fund,* we were able to weather the difficulties cancer imposed on our lives and came out the other side even more inspired.

A note about the cancer fund: What my husband learned through all of this is how little financial assistance is available for men or male breadwinners when they get cancer. And, it can be devastating financially for the whole family when the breadwinner gets ill. Knowing this, we created our *Cancer Recovery Fund* to help us pay our cancer-related medical bills, and it was a lifesaver!

One final note about paying your medical bills. You never know where help will come from. Just stay open to the possibilities. One of my husband's friends who owns a nightclub generously offered to give my husband a benefit to help raise money for the fund. Anything is possible. Think big!

Chapter 12

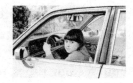

The Feeding Tube Rumba

As I mentioned in the General Advice section, if your doctor recommends a feeding tube, if at all possible, make sure the patient has the feeding tube surgery done early in the process. While the patient probably won't need to eat by feeding tube for a few weeks, they will have an easier time of recuperating from the feeding tube surgery while they are still capable of eating by mouth rather than later in the process when they may need to be using the feeding tube exclusively for nourishing and staying hydrated.

In my husband's case, because he continued to eat by mouth until his 6th week of cancer treatments *(yes - this is quite unusual)* - he used the tube for extra hydration *(water and juices)* during most of his treatment weeks. He also used the tube to feed himself liquid nutrition for about the last week of cancer treatments and for an additional couple of weeks after the cancer treatments were finished while he slowly reintegrated regular food back into his life.

What can I say besides *"Having a feeding tube is really not a very pleasant experience?"* In my husband's case, we opted to have the procedure done during the first week of chemo and radiation. My husband's feeding tube surgery required an overnight stay in the hospital and an overnight stay for me at a nearby hotel. John needed downtime to recover and there was definitely a learning curve in figuring out how to properly use the feeding tube, keep it clean, etc.

Not knowing anything about feeding tubes, we were ill prepared for the whole process. I remember being in shock sitting at my husband's bedside at the hospital the day after my husband's operation. A perky nutritionist dressed in a business suit and high heels was sent in before checkout to demonstrate how to use the feeding tube for nourishment and hydration. While she had a *"captive audience,"* my husband was barely alert, trying to sit up in bed and pay attention, as if he was taking a crash course in a foreign language. I watched the demo with a combination of amusement, annoyance, and horror. The *"class"* went on for nearly two hours and my husband was not to be discharged until he had met with the nutritionist and received his feeding tube lesson. I remember asking her, *"Isn't there a video of your demo so we can watch it when my husband isn't so drugged up?"* *"No,"* she answered. *"But that's a great idea."* And I kept thinking, "OHMYGOD ... is this real?"

Of course, a bubbly nutritionist waving and flexing the demo feeding tube in the air and into a small can of liquid food from across the room is not quite the same as trying to feed a frightened loved one who is in pain and despair. After checkout, the nutritionist insisted on following me to my car while wheeling an overwhelming stack of tools and equipment for us to bring home, including: cases of canned, liquid nutrition; bandages; a pole for gravity feeding *(if needed)*; plastic syringes for measuring liquid food and inserting into the feeding tube; and long, cotton swabs for cleaning the skin around the feeding tube. I know she was just doing her job, but we did feel forced into taking all that stuff home, even though we were uncertain that we'd ever use most of it. I asked the nutritionist if her company could deliver the equipment to our home and could she come to our house to do the demo instead, but she said, *"No."* Her job was to teach my husband at the hospital and that was that.

Based on what the surgeon had told us, we expected a speedy recovery where my husband would be up and about the next day. But no such luck. My hubbie was doubled-up in pain and spent the entire weekend in bed. It took him the better part of a week to begin to feel like he could walk, sit, and move about relatively normally - and he was very angry about having to have a feeding tube at all. He couldn't imagine he'd ever need to use it. I did my best to be cool about it. And we were both very glad toward the end of treatment that he had a feeding tube installed. If he hadn't had one, he couldn't have eaten at all for several weeks, and that would have been devastating.

As for using the tube, if you have any questions, just ask your doctor. We found that the nurses were more than happy to help my husband feed himself during his doctor visits or chemo sessions. They all know how to do it. You should also be provided with written instructions on care, usage, cleaning, etc. Most of the time my husband had his feeding tube he managed to be able to use it, feed himself, clean it, and take care of it by himself. We did have a few *"scares,"* however. One was early on when the tube stuck to the surrounding skin. It was a Sunday and we didn't know what to do. Our family physician was an angel and called us immediately to let us know the condition was very common and not to worry. He had my husband basically twirl the feeding tube to loosen it a bit and told him he needed to turn it every so often so it wouldn't stick. Thankfully, this problem never happened again.

Removing the feeding tube was a heck of a lot easier than installing it. Removal involved a brief outpatient visit, a small bandage with a few cursory instructions for care and cleaning, and away we went. Feeding tubes do create permanent scars, but other than that, there have been no residual problems.

Here are a few feeding tube tips:
For leaking: The feeding tube did leak early on. If you don't mind ooey-gooey things, great. Otherwise, it's quite gross, but nothing that requires a professional cleaning service. I'm just kidding! It might be a bit bloody, and it might leak stomach contents. There - I said it. If it stains clothes or bedding, have some hydrogen peroxide on hand. Otherwise, a warm, wet washcloth should do the trick. Bring extra bandages and tape with you when you are out in the world, in case you have to change the feeding tube bandages that lay over the tube on top of the skin. And, if the patient is a side-sleeper, it's going to be messy at first, but the messiness should subside in a few weeks.

For food temperature: Be sure the food is neither ice cold or hot. Remember - the food is being directly poured into the stomach, so extremes in temperature can be painful. Room temp or slightly warm is best.

For food consistency: Make sure the food is smooth and relatively thin. Think: watery and watered down. And, definitely nothing sticky, chunky, pebbly, or syrupy, or you'll have a devil of a time cleaning the tube.

Cleaning: There are various methods for cleaning the tube. We found that just flushing it before and after meals with room temperature water was fine. My husband used the tube for adding extra water and staying hydrated throughout the day, so the tube stayed fairly clean. The nutritionist suggested tonic water and meat tenderizer. This gave me *"the willies."* If you need something stronger than water, ask your doctor what they suggest.

Fashion: You're thinking, *"What does fashion have to do with this?"* Well - the feeding tube protrudes from the stomach and shows through clothes. We solved this problem by buying black t-shirts and black shirts that were not too fitted, and this seemed to do the trick for the most part. Dressing in layers, with an outer shirt or open jacket over black or dark colors can hide the tube, as well. If not, tell people your loved one just won the Guinness World Book of Records for *"the biggest outie."* Just kidding, but you get the point. You might as well have fun with it and get a good laugh!

Chapter 13

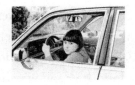

What to Ask Your Doctor

This is an important time to get educated about what's going on and what to expect. The more you know, the better equipped you'll be to handle the ups and downs of what lies ahead. Unless you work in a cancer treatment facility or have helped others through this situation, you can't possibly be prepared for what's in store. We certainly were not, which is one reason I wrote this book. While we were given a few info sheets from various doctors, what was written on those pages was... well... *"Cancer Lite"* compared to what really ended up happening to my husband. As a result, we were always scrambling to try to figure out what was going on and how to fix things. It doesn't have to be this way for you.

When selecting your medical team, make sure your primary oncologist is experienced in dealing with your particular type of cancer and is staying *"in the know"* on the latest and greatest protocols and procedures. Don't be afraid to ask how many cases they've seen and what the results were. Your medical team needs to inspire trust and gain your confidence. If you have any doubts about their level of expertise, trust your instincts and move on.

Your doctor will be your main resource for all your questions. Don't be afraid to speak up and ask questions. No question should be too big or too small. If they don't know the answer, they can point you to those who do, whether it's other practitioners, books, web sites, etc. Just ask! Ask for information about the various studies being done, the protocols they will administer, and why they're necessary. One of the things I learned after the fact was that in the western medicine arena there is consensus worldwide about what the most effective course of treatment is for throat cancer. So there is plenty of data out there if you're interested in learning more - especially before treatment begins. I also learned that in other parts of the world, throat cancer patients are as *"in the dark"* as we were about what to expect and what to do at home to take care of our loved ones. Another reason why I wrote this book!

Understand that today's science is tomorrow's science fiction, and vice versa. As we learn more, study more, and understand more, protocols and procedures get changed and rearranged. Doctors are not gods but they are often scholars. And, they are relying on the evidence from studies being done by others in their field. Ask questions. In addition, cancer is big business for the clinics, hospitals, drug companies, and everyone involved in the process, including the canned nutrition manufacturers. So, it's healthy to question why you need things, what they're for, what the results will be, and what the alternatives are.

Here are some questions to ask your doctor(s):

1. What is the protocol you'll be using to cure my throat cancer? What are the pros and cons of using this protocol?
2. What should I expect in the way of symptoms and side effects and how will you be dealing with them?

3. What are the best case/worst case scenarios for my type of cancer? *(Tell it to me straight, doc.)*
4. What will you be recommending for pain management?
5. How can I reach you if there's an emergency or a severe change in my symptoms?
6. Will you be here for my entire cancer treatment or are you planning to be out of town at all? If you'll be leaving, who will be taking over for you in your absence? Can I meet them before I begin treatment?
7. What tests will I need to take and when? What are the risks and potential side effects of these tests?
8. Can I have a tour of the facility? Can I see the room where I will be receiving chemo treatments? Can I see the room where I will be receiving radiation?
9. Can I wait a few weeks or a month before I begin treatments so that I can reorganize my life and get things in order?

Questions to ask your doctor on a weekly basis *(or more, if symptoms are concerning to you)*:

1. Am I on track?
2. Are any of the symptoms better or worse than you expected?
3. What can I expect in the coming week?

In general, if something doesn't look right, feel right, or isn't going well, speak up. For instance, if you're not comfortable on the radiation table before you begin *(too hot, cold, etc.)* ask for whatever you need. Get comfortable. If you need a blanket or a pillow for your knees, just ask. You'll be expected to lay perfectly still on the treatment table for 20-30 minutes and you should not be in pain or discomfort during this procedure. In fact, the scary thing is that it doesn't hurt while you're getting radiation, yet the effects are intense, shocking, and potentially destructive to other things beside your cancer (*e.g., your thyroid*).

Above all - speak up if anything seems wrong. If you aren't happy with one nurse, ask for another. And, unless you're at a training facility, you do not have to give your consent to be used for observation and training new staff members. Your privacy is a right, not a privilege.

Chapter 14

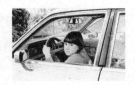

Ever-Changing Symptoms, Side Effects, and What to Expect

Symptoms are ever-changing - especially during treatment - and vary widely from patient to patient. Just as you think you've got a handle on things, they'll change. What worked one day didn't work the next. Sometimes my husband's symptoms changed hour by hour. For us, dealing with ever-changing symptoms was confusing, frustrating, and often alarming. It was especially stressful to not understand what was happening or what to expect down the road. And, we were definitely not prepared to deal with many of the scariest symptoms. So, here's a *"heads up"* about what might be in store for you. As always, check with your medical team to discuss symptoms and side effects and to learn the best ways to treat them.

Symptoms my husband experienced before he was diagnosed with throat cancer:

- An earache that came and went

- A sore throat that came and went

- Difficulty swallowing

- Salivary gland infection that never fully healed
- Swollen glands
- Weight loss

Symptoms my husband experienced during his treatment regime:

- Acid stomach
- Allergic reaction to medicine causing all-over body rash
- Anxiety
- Change in ability to taste foods, i.e., food either tastes strange or has no flavor at all
- Coughing
- Depression
- Difficulty swallowing
- Dry mouth
- Earache
- Exhaustion
- Fevers
- Hoarse or froggy-sounding voice
- Inability to sleep
- Low stamina/endurance
- Mood swings
- Muscular weakness
- Nasal congestion
- Nausea
- Needing to clear the throat and spit

- Physically cold *(even in summer)*
- Runny, drippy nose *(and food can come out the nose when sneezing - yikes!)*
- Severe burn on neck and face - very red with skin peeling, sloughing off, and oozing
- Severe, localized pain
- Snoring *(like a wild boar!)*
- Sores in the mouth and on the tongue
- Sore throat
- Sun-sensitivity *(extreme)*
- Swollen lymph glands
- The need for more rest during the day and more sleep at night
- Voice sounding lower than normal
- Weight loss

A year and a half after being cancer-free, here are the symptoms my husband still experiences:

- A residual *"pouch"* below his chin where the cancer was located
- Dry mouth *(but improving)*
- Manufacturing a minimal amount of saliva; needing liquids to help swallow foods
- Occasional coughing - especially when eating anything dry, doughy, or seedy
- Sun sensitivity *(especially face and neck)*
- Difficulty staying warm; needing extra layers of clothing during the day and extra blankets at night

- Minimal weight gain *(regained 12 out of the 35 pounds lost)*
- Needing to keep immune system strong
- Voice still lower than normal, especially when tired
- The need for extra sleep and the need to sleep later in the morning
- The need to keep the pace very moderate at work
- The need to live a relatively low-paced, stress-free life

A few things to expect before, during, and after treatment:

Positioning mask and mouth guard:
Before treatment begins, the radiation team will create a special positioning mask custom-made to fit your face. It is a special mold designed to keep the head stationary during treatments that will be bolted to the radiation table to perfectly line up the radiation beams to the right spots each time. Each week there will be a re-calibration of the positioning mask to make sure the head is still lined up properly during treatments.

The radiation team will also create a custom mouth guard that you will wear during radiation treatments to protect your teeth and mouth. Metal fillings can create radiation *"scatter"* in the mouth that can cause painful mouth sores and swelling. If you have any metal fillings or crowns, consider having them replaced with ceramic fillings before you begin treatment.

The positioning mask and the mouth guard may feel weird, but they should not hurt. If you are experiencing any pain, speak up!

About pain management:
Pain management is an important part of the treatment process. One of the radiation treatment techs warned my husband not to let pain get out of control, as the throat cancer protocol is considered to be one of the most severe radiation protocols for any type of cancer he performs. This turned out to be excellent advice.

About mouth sores:
In addition to your oncologist, call your dentist if you develop mouth sores. Our dentist was able to provide relief for my husband and helped speed up his healing by giving him a particular mouthwash that killed specific oral bacteria.

A note about chemo:
Some facilities administer chemo to patients in a group setting. While it might be a more social experience depending on who is next to you, it can also be distressing to see so many people suffering. Make it your choice whether or not to have a private room. If your center doesn't offer privacy and that is something you want, choose another facility.

After treatment:
You will probably be sent to a speech therapist to learn swallowing exercises and to make sure you are swallowing correctly. You will probably also be sent to a physical therapist to be given exercises for regaining strength and rebuilding muscle mass from all the weight loss.

Follow-up visits and tests:
There will be follow-up visits with your oncology team over the next year or more. And, there will also be more blood tests, scans, etc. - to ensure you are cancer-free. If all goes well and you are cancer-free a year after treatment ends, you can expect to be done with those dreadful tests - yay!

Chapter 15

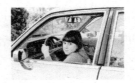

Mommy Medicine

There's Western Medicine, Eastern Medicine, and what I call *"Mommy Medicine."* No - it's not a technical term. I made it up and speak of it often. Here's what it means: While all the other doctors are busy poking, prodding, testing, examining, analyzing, and treating - mommy is the one who is observing her family members on a daily basis and in some ways, sees much more than the doctors can in the little time they have with the patient. Mommies notice when our family members don't look right, sound right, etc. Little imperceptible changes that others may not notice can cause alarm bells to go off for Mommy. Mommies use their intuition and navigate with their hearts. Mommy medicine is all the things we do at home to help our loved ones heal and stay healthy. It's the nurturing, caring, loving, and caretaking that can make all the difference between sickness and health. This is Mommy Medicine. It is neither male nor female. It just is.

Never underestimate the power and importance Mommy Medicine plays in helping to get the throat cancer patient well. While the oncologists are busy doing everything they can to save your loved one's life, they don't live with the patient, sit next to them on the sofa and watch movies with them, share meals with them, drive them to and from their doctor appointments, or listen to them breathing while they sleep. Your observations, experiences, and questions may very well provide the missing pieces to making your loved one whole again.

In addition, Mommy Medicine may include cleaning wounds, administering salves and ointments to tender, painful skin, changing bandages, and providing endless amounts of patience during emotionally challenging times. This is invaluable. Before treatment began, I remember telling my husband's doctors that I was not the nursing type and that I had no desire to deal with *"ooey-gooey things."* But somehow in spite of myself, I found the fortitude to deal with it all and the unshakeable will to support my husband, *"ooey-gooeyness"* and all.

Rising to the occasion and doing a great job can be rewarding in and of itself. Remember to pat yourself on the back for a job well done. Don't expect to be thanked much for providing great Mommy Medicine. Unfortunately, Mommies/caregivers are often overlooked in the whole healing process. In fact, Mommies can be treated rather invisibly during the treatment phase, as doctors and their staff are focused on getting the patient well. At the end of treatment, don't be shy about asking for a round of applause from the oncology team. You deserve it!

Chapter 16

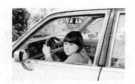

The Emotional Side
of Throat Cancer

Whether you're a patient or caregiver, dealing with throat cancer can be a crazy-making ordeal. Welcome to the *Emotional Olympics!* Hey - while you're at it, aim for the Gold!

This is a wacky time. Your life is going along perfectly well and then WHAMMO! Just like that, everything is turned upside down. Life as you know it has changed. If you're the patient, your needs, daily routines, and ability to work are in flux. Your ability to be independent, strong, and take care of others? Gone. Just when you think you have things under control, BLAMMO. Back to square one. Self-confidence can easily be replaced by fear, confusion, irritability, and anger. And while you're at it, throw in a healthy dose of outrage, a dash of grief, and a big fat scoop of overwhelm. You are understandably upset. After all, you didn't plan for this to happen. Who would?

So life has thrown you a major curve ball. While you didn't expect or set out to deal with throat cancer right now, how you react to and deal with it are critical elements for your emotional wellbeing. Hi. You've just entered a life-threatening, real-life drama. Now, act normal. But wait - what is normal? Time to create a new normal with new strategies for coping with and getting through this wacky time. You'll need to muster up all your physical and emotional reserves to get through this - and then some. Seeing the pain and suffering that your loved one is undergoing can be emotionally heartwrenching. And it can be challenging at times to just stay focused and *"keep calm and carry on,"* as they say. But you can do it!

For the caregiver and the patient, one strategy is to *"suck it up"* and just power through the whole experience. You'll be so busy taking care of things and dealing with various crises you never dreamed of, you won't have too much time to indulge in your feelings. But when you do have time it would be a good idea to talk things out with someone who can be compassionate about your experience. Whether it's a trusted friend or family member, someone who's gone through this before and come out the other side, a therapist, or a support group *(or all of the above)*, please make sure you create opportunities to express what's going on for you.

If you don't deal with what's happening emotionally while you're going through it, I can guarantee you'll pay a price for this down the road. I chose the *"power through it all"* strategy, which kept me going strong until a few months after my husband finished treatment. But my husband's cancer took its toll on me, too - and I needed more healing and rejuvenation than I realized. For the next 9 months or so, I felt exhausted, depleted, and in dire need of recuperation physically and emotionally. The drama and the trauma of nearly losing my husband to cancer was stressful, to say the least. I had to be strong not only for my husband, but also for our kids, our families, for running our business, and keeping us afloat financially. I was the primary decision-maker for everything, as my husband was in many ways incapacitated. Often I had to deal with, confront, and solve all our difficulties and challenges by myself. While I rose to the occasion and found a reservoir of strength I didn't know was there, it didn't last forever and I definitely had to take time to take care of me, too.

At the clinics I remember seeing signs for *"free yoga class"* or *"free massage"* for the cancer patients. And I thought, *"Hey - what about me?"* Fortunately, there were many opportunities for the patient to receive nurturing and emotional support through the cancer clinics. But the caregivers were a rather invisible group whose needs were only minimally addressed by the clinics. There were no specific support groups for caregivers who were dealing with throat cancer. All cancers were lumped into one. Hopefully, that will change.

Bearing in mind that the oncology centers are primarily designed to serve the patients and not the caregivers, be sure to think about what would be nurturing and healing for you and then make time to do it. The key is this: if you create healthy opportunities to express yourself and nurture yourself *away from* the patient, you won't end up feeling resentful or angry *with* the patient. After all, your life has been turned upside down, too. But it *will* get better. Just hang in there!

For tips and advice on de-stressing and getting through this tumultuous time, see the chapters on Staying Sane and Seeing the Humor.

Chapter 17

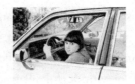

Home Remedies
for Symptom Relief

Many years ago, I discovered a number of home remedies for a variety of common symptoms and I usually keep these remedies on hand *"just in case."* In our experience, these home remedies came in quite handy for helping with my husband's healing process during throat cancer, as well. The only new formula was *Orithrush*, which was specific to symptoms my husband experienced only during his cancer treatments.

The following home remedies are not meant to be a substitute for cancer treatments, prescribed medicine, etc. They are simply meant to be helpful tools to have on hand at home, if needed. As always, be sure to check with your doctors to make sure you don't administer any lotions, potions, vitamins, or formulas that could conflict with the patient's treatment regime.

For information about specific products and brands that we personally use, be sure to check out my Resources chapter.

Aloe Vera Gel & Vitamin E
What's it for: This is a wonderful topical ointment for burns, sunburns, etc. It is soothing, healing, and should not be painful.

Because I have allergies to chemical fragrances and perfumes, my husband rejected the chemically fragranced salves the doctors initially provided for him. The aloe & E combo, with its neutral fragrance, proved to be a wonderful alternative to the perfumed salves. We found aloe & E to be especially useful in the early weeks of treatment and then again after treatments were completed.

How to: Mix a few drops of vitamin E oil into a tablespoon of aloe vera gel. Vitamin E is available in capsules by the bottle or in a dropper bottle *(in the vitamin section of your grocery store)*. If you use the capsules, just cut open a few capsules and squeeze the oil out. Or, squeeze a dropper of vitamin E oil into the tablespoon of aloe vera gel. Make sure both the aloe and the vitamin E are as pure as possible, i.e., free of chemical ingredients or preservatives. This wonderful mixture can be smoothed onto the radiated neck and face area several times a day.

Aloe Vera Juice

What's it for: Drinking Aloe Vera juice can be soothing, cooling, and healing to the digestive tract, mucosal tissues, etc. It may help with the *"sunburn inside the throat"* caused by radiation treatments for throat cancer. I had my husband drink 2 ounces of juice, two to three times per day. Maybe this was coincidental, but my husband did not suffer from pain in his throat during throat cancer treatments, which I understand is quite unusual. While I can't say for sure that it was the aloe juice, we believe it certainly helped.

How to: The Aloe Vera juice one drinks is a completely different product than the gel one uses topically, so be sure you understand what you're buying. When using aloe juice, measure out a few ounces and swish and swallow the juice by itself. Do not mix with or follow right away with any other foods, beverages, or medicines. It coats the throat with a soothing, healing liquid. Most aloe juices need to be refrigerated after opening so be sure to read the labels. Also - not all aloe juices taste the same. Some aloe juices taste a bit bitter and medicinal, while others are much more neutral tasting or pleasant. For our favorite brands, see the resource chapter.

Digestive Enzymes
What's it for: Digestive enzymes are necessary for breaking down proteins, fats, and carbohydrates to help us not only digest foods but to absorb nutrients, as well. While we naturally manufacture these enzymes, some people need extra help digesting - and as we age, many of us don't manufacture as many digestive enzymes as we need.

Digestion begins in the mouth with saliva being the first process to help break down food so it can be absorbed. During radiation treatments for throat cancer, the salivary glands can be greatly affected and can stop producing the volume of saliva needed to begin digesting food. In our experience, this is where digestive enzymes were a great help.

How to: Digestive enzymes can be found at most health food stores, vitamin shops, or vitamin stores online. You do not need a prescription for them. Most digestive enzymes come in pill form, but you can also find them as a liquid or powder. Follow the instructions on the manufacturer's label, as there are many different brands and they have different directions. Most digestive enzymes are taken just before eating a meal. Some are taken after a meal, especially if they include ingredients like peppermint or papaya. If swallowing pills is difficult, put the pills in a spoonful of applesauce. Applesauce coats the pill and makes it much easier to swallow.

Make sure the formula includes enzymes that help break down protein, carbohydrates, and fat *(amylase, protease, and lipase)*. Some digestive enzyme formulas contain animal products such as Pancreatin. If you prefer not to eat animal products, there are many vegetarian products available. I've been taking digestive enzyme supplements for many years now - and so has my husband. In our experience, we have definitely noticed an improvement in our ability to digest foods. For suggestions on brands, check the resource chapter. And be sure to ask your doctor if it's ok to take them.

Note: If you have heartburn or acid reflux, do not take any formulas containing HCL *(hydrochloric acid)*. HCL can create more acid, which only exacerbates the problem.

Salt Water Rinses
What's it for: Rinsing the mouth and throat with a mild, salty solution can be helpful in killing bacteria and soothing open sores *(canker sores, etc.)*. This can be especially helpful with mouth sores - which are a common side effect of throat cancer treatments.

How to: Dissolve ½ teaspoon of sea salt in a glass of room temperature water *(6-8 oz.)*. Stir the mixture to make sure the salt is evenly distributed. Swish the salty water around the mouth, gargle, and spit it out. Repeat until all the salt water is used up. You can do this treatment several times per day.

Ginger Tea
What's it for: Ginger is a time-honored remedy for nausea and tummy upsets.

How to: Ginger is available as either a root, in tea bags, or dried with a sugar coating. To balance out nausea, I prefer drinking ginger tea. In purchasing tea, look for a brand that has only one ingredient: ginger. Many companies mix ginger with all kinds of ingredients, including black pepper - which is not something you'll want at this time. You can also make a tea by boiling the ginger root *(available in the veggie section of your grocery store)*. To use the root, peel a couple of inches of ginger root and place in a pot with several cups of water. Bring to a boil - then simmer for 20 minutes or so. Strain out the ginger root and enjoy. A note of caution: be careful with ginger tea, as it is warming. Drink it no hotter than room temp - and use this only in the early stages of treatment. Once the radiation is beginning to inflame the throat tissues, ginger may be too warm, so use your best judgment on this.

Wellness Formulas
What's it for: Wellness formulas are used as preventatives for colds and flu. In my experience, when taken at the first sign of a cold or virus, wellness formulas can often knock out the bug and prevent you from getting sick. These formulas usually contain a variety of herbal and/or homeopathic ingredients known for boosting the immune system.

How to: At the first sign of a cold or flu, follow the dosage recommended by the manufacturer. Make sure you read the label and rule out allergies to any of the ingredients before using. Golden Seal, for example, is not good for people with ragweed allergies. Wellness formulas would be great to have on hand for use before and well after the cancer treatment regime is over. Check with your doctor to make sure there aren't any ingredients that conflict with their treatment regimes. I am not recommending the use of wellness *(immune-boosting)* formulas during chemo and radiation. These formulas can be used to build up a weakened immune system before treatment - and then later on a few months after treatment is over, as needed.

Tri-Salts

What's it for: Tri-Salts is one of my favorite formulas that I keep on hand. I also bring it with me whenever I'm traveling. It is an alkalinizing formula that balances out an acid stomach and is fast-acting. Tri-Salts are sodium-free and contain calcium carbonate, magnesium carbonate, and potassium carbonate. My husband loved this product and found it to be very effective in combatting the acid stomach and acid reflux that chemo and radiation produced.

How to: Tri-Salts is a powder. When you have an acid stomach, dissolve ½ - 1 teaspoon of Tri-Salts in a small glass of water. Stir and drink the solution. You should notice relief in ten to fifteen minutes. Tri-Salts are made by Ecological Formulas, listed in my resource chapter. You can order directly from the company and they are wonderful to deal with.

Orithrush

What's it for: Orithrush is a mouth rinse used for treating oral Thrush - a fungal infection of the mouth and tongue. On visual inspection, Thrush looks like a furry, white coating on the tongue. For the cancer patient, Chemo and radiation can be the culprits behind a stubborn case of Thrush. We were at our wit's end trying to get rid of the Thrush and tried a variety of prescriptions, but to no avail. In our experience, once my husband tried Orithrush, his symptoms began to diminish.

How to: Orithrush is a concentrated liquid that you mix with water, one dose at a time. It is used as a mouth rinse and gargle in much the same way a salt-water rinse for canker sores would be used. Follow the instructions on the Orithrush label. And, if you have any questions, just call the company *(Ecological Formulas - listed in our resource chapter).*

Chapter 18

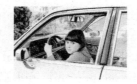

Getting the Best Nutrition
or ... *shake shake shake!*

One of the best things you can do for the throat cancer patient is to help them get the nutrition they need. Your loved one will need to consume many more calories than they normally need, and this is an adjustment that requires planning, preparation, and lots of patience. Most patients will be given cases of high-calorie, liquid nutrition as canned drinks that are covered by most health insurance plans. While the prevailing theory is *"just pack on the calories"* - and the canned nutritional drinks are most certainly an easy way, if you have the time and motivation to prepare healthy foods, it will pay off in great dividends later on. First, there's nothing to compare to the nutritional value we get from eating wholesome fresh fruits, vegetables, proteins, and grains. Since my husband and I usually eat a very healthy diet comprised of mainly fresh, organic, home-cooked meals, my husband's digestive system was quite simply not used to eating processed, canned foods and after ingesting one can of liquid nutrition provided by the hospital's nutritionist, he immediately got indigestion. He was miserable. So for us, it was not a choice. To keep my husband's system as happy and healthy as it could be throughout the whole cancer ordeal, I had to continue making healthy meals for him in whatever form he could most easily tolerate. Fortunately for my husband, I like to cook and am a pretty good cook as well - so coming up with yummy, high calorie, healthy foods was not a problem for me. I actually enjoyed it. When my husband was well enough, he followed my recipes and cooked for himself. Here are some tips and guidelines for making the best foods and best choices possible:

Things that work

The easiest way to get the most calories is to drink them. I made high-calorie/high nutrition smoothies, soups, and desserts that were easy to swallow. Think silky, smooth, liquid, and creamy. Think cool, slightly warm, or room temperature. Think mashed, pureed, soupy, ground fine, melt in your mouth, simple, easy to swallow, easy to digest foods. Think baby food consistency, juicy, nectars. Think comfort food that is mushy, like mashed potatoes and gravy.

Things to avoid

Your loved one will probably not be able to manufacture enough saliva to break down food, will most likely complain of *"dry mouth,"* and might suffer from mouth sores. Additionally, they may have pain in their throat whenever they swallow. Therefore, avoid foods that are crunchy, dry, hard, sharp-edged, or crispy. Avoid doughy textures and foods that require lots of saliva and liquids to be swallowed. Avoid hot or extreme temperatures in food and avoid anything spicy, peppery, citrus, or acidic, as these will burn the mouth and throat. Avoid foods that are tough, chewy, stringy, fibrous, gummy, or pasty. Also avoid foods that contain seeds and nuts in whole form. Avoid large chunks of food or any foods that require lots of chewing in order to swallow.

Adding more calories

Because I usually think in terms of slimming my meals down and deleting the foods that add extra calories and fat, I had to do the reverse of everything I'd always done - and this was a challenge at first. My husband's nutritionist had initially told us that he needed to eat 2,300 calories per day. But she had substantially misjudged his intake needs. By trial and error, we discovered my husband needed to eat - *drum roll please* - **4,000** calories a day in order to not lose weight. I'm not kidding! It can be a challenge to eat that many calories per day, as there's only so much that a person can digest at any given time, with or without a feeding tube. Hence, sneaking in extra calories here and there can make a huge difference. Here are some ideas that worked for us:

Add calories with a serving or two of healthy oil to each meal. Oils such as sesame, olive, etc., can be added to soups with little difference in taste. Adding a tablespoon of sesame, olive, or coconut oil to whatever you're cooking is an easy way to add another 120 calories. Look for *Extra Virgin* or *Unrefined* oils as they have more food value than refined.

Add calories by including coconut in your meals. Coconut has wonderful nutritional and healing benefits and packs a lot of calories, to boot. Although it has gotten a bad rap over the years, coconut is enjoying a bit of resurgence right now. While cow's milk and dairy can contribute to the production of inflammation and congestion in some people, coconut has anti-inflammatory properties and even anti-fungal properties. I added coconut wherever I could, including frozen coconut desserts to smoothies *(a yummy alternative to ice cream)*, warm coconut oil to smoothies, coconut milk to soups and sauces, and coconut oil in lieu of butter to brownies and other treats. In addition, the frozen coconut desserts we added to smoothies were sweetened with agave, which is low on the *Glycemic Index* and doesn't spike one's blood sugar the way regular sugar does. When buying coconut oil, look for *"extra virgin,"* as it tends to have more nutrients.

Add calories with plain, salt-free nuts. Finely grind the nuts and add them to smoothies, desserts, etc. As an example, ½ cup of walnuts is almost 400 calories and is loaded with nutrients, yet it does not increase the volume of a smoothie very much.

Add calories with creamy, ripe avocados, which are loaded with good oils and beneficial nutrients.

Add extra calories with apple juice and other fruit juices. Glasses of apple juice throughout the day help with hydration as well as adding extra calories. In general, fruit juices have 100-120 calories per glass. My husband was able to drink 4 glasses of juice per day, which easily added 400 - 500 calories to his daily regime. I bought organic apple juice by the gallon. You can also buy juice in individual boxes for travel that need no refrigeration. And, juices are easy to come by whenever the patient is out and about. Even convenience stores carry them.

While we started with plain fruit juices, later on in John's treatment process, he found thicker nectars to be easier to swallow than straight juices. Try nectars such as mango, pear, peach, and apricot. And, be sure to avoid any acidic fruits or fruit juices, as they can be quite painful to swallow and can sting the raw tissues in the mouth and throat. Ouch!

Add calories with dairy products, if the patient isn't allergic to them. Add a few tablespoons of sour cream or yogurt to a cup of soup; add cream to soups and chowders; and be guilt-free about adding ice cream or other frozen desserts to smoothies, desserts, and milk shakes. Milk shakes are great for adding more calories and can be fun to eat. One of our friends came to visit and brought my husband a big milk shake. The visit cheered my husband up and the milk shake gave him hundreds of enjoyable extra calories that day.

Other tips
Incorporate bananas into your daily smoothies. Bananas are high in potassium, which gets depleted during chemo. Bananas each day keep potassium deficiencies at bay. A little levity.

Make soups, soups, and more soups. I made big vats of things and pureed them or semi-pureed them, and filled the freezer with containers of soup. Alternatively, you can freeze pureed soups in ice cube trays, as they are easier to defrost that way. Check out my recipe section for ideas on soups you can make.

Make a daily smoothie. The smoothie I made for my husband varied somewhat from day to day, but incorporated the following: soy milk or rice milk *(you can also use almond milk or cow's milk)*, bananas and a variety of fresh and frozen fruit, protein powder, coconut oil, lecithin, ground nuts, and ground flax seeds. You can make several servings and refrigerate the rest. Smoothies are quite portable and easy to carry on the road in a thermos. They can also be heated slightly, or thinned down, as needed. And, smoothies can easily add 500 - 2,500 calories per day. See my recipe section for ideas.

Get an A+ in pureeing. You can basically puree or mash just about any cooked food *(well - almost)*. Just try it. If you add enough liquid and whiz it up in a blender, it will eventually become smooth and creamy. Think of it as making your own homemade baby food with any veggies you steam up, any fruits you cook, or even cooked meats and fish. You can certainly take your loved one's favorite meals and simply puree them *(like lasagna)*, but not everything will taste or look right when you do. Meals with many colors can turn grey or brown when you puree everything together. And, for the person undergoing throat cancer treatments, it's hard enough to muster up the desire to eat, let alone the desire to eat something that looks awful. My advice: rather than putting the entire dinner in the blender, try pureeing foods with similar colors and serving them separately. It'll cut down on the *"yuck"* factor.

Make sure the patient isn't allergic to any of the foods you're preparing. And, by all means, if anything seems to cause digestive problems, eliminate them immediately. Also - be sure to ask your doctor if any of the foods or nutritional supplements you are using could negatively interact with or delay the effectiveness of their treatment regimes or medicines they administer for throat cancer.

Add "cooling" foods to meals and snacks. Cooling foods can be beneficial, especially if it's not the dead of winter in a cold climate when your loved one is undergoing treatment. In Chinese medicine, cooling foods such as tofu, cucumber, and watermelon are beneficial for cooling down the system, especially during radiation (*i.e., "hot"*) treatments.

Buy lecithin granules and add to smoothies. Lecithin is great for calming frayed nerves and helps with digesting fats and assimilating fat-soluble vitamins. We used two tablespoons per day in smoothies.

Consider incorporating preservative-free aloe juice into the patient's daily regime. Aloe is soothing, healing, and great for the digestive tract, as well. I had my husband drink about 2 ounces, 2-3 times per day. Don't mix it in with anything. Just have your loved one drink it by itself. Drinking aloe juice upon arising and at bedtime may prove beneficial for healing the tissues of the mouth and throat, as aloe is a time-honored remedy for healing burns and sunburns. Taken internally, it may help soothe the *"sunburn in the throat"* that many throat cancer patients experience due to radiation treatments. Make sure you are buying food grade aloe juice for drinking. Aloe gel is not the same thing and should only be used externally. For suggestions of which brands of aloe juice to buy, see my resource chapter at the end of the book.

Try putting pills in a spoonful of applesauce to help them go down, since vitamin tablets and other pills will undoubtedly be hard to swallow. You can also crush pills and put them in applesauce, as well. With all the irritation and inflammation in the throat, pills can get caught on their way down, even when swallowing with plenty of water or juice. Alternatively, buy vitamins in liquid form, as they'll be much easier to swallow and digest. But be sure liquid vitamins don't have anything in them that could burn, such as pineapple or citrus.

Use yummy smells to entice your loved one to eat. During cancer treatments, the patient can often have their sense of taste change, diminish, or go away entirely - at least temporarily. This is quite common. With some sense of humor we called it *"eating in black and white."* Since taste is only one facet of the enjoyment of eating, I came up with a neat trick to get my husband to be more motivated to eat. Here's what to do: before a meal, ask the patient to close their eyes and then smell the food. Their sense of smell should still be intact - and smelling the food, especially if it has yummy ingredients - may help entice them to eat. Try it!

Make sure there is nothing impeding the patient's ability to eat. Sometimes the patient may not want to complain. In one instance, my husband suddenly couldn't swallow a smoothie I'd made for him that had fresh strawberries. I didn't realize that the strawberry seeds were getting caught in my husband's throat and making him cough, which was quite painful. I whisked the smoothie away and pushed the smoothie mixture through a sieve, thereby eliminating the strawberry seeds. It only took a few minutes and made a world of difference.

Take the patient out for a meal or snack. Early on in my husband's treatment, I made it a habit to take him out for a latté or a small meal several times a week. We often went to a cafe after radiation sessions. My husband is a very social guy and it helped his morale to be out and about, even though at one point he looked like *"the invisible man"* with bandages around his neck covered with a colorful bandana. I'd say to him, *"Just pick something on the menu and try it."* And he would. We discovered he could eat scrambled eggs, pancakes and syrup, breakfast sausages, fruit blintzes, various soups, sometimes a pasta dish, and many foods served with gravies and sauces. Even if he could only take a few bites after mashing up the food on his plate, it made him feel normal and helped him feel successful. And, of course, it helped me to feel successful, too. It isn't easy being a full-time cheerleader and those little successes are very important all around.

Chapter 19

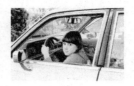

Go Ahead -
Have the Brownie!

While I'm all for eating healthy and taking good care of yourself, this is not the time to hold back on enjoying simple pleasures. If this phase of your life teaches you nothing else, you should be realizing by now that life is fragile, precious, and fleeting. Living in the moment and savoring things should be on your agenda right now. Seize a few special moments here and there to enjoy life.

The smell of warm chocolate baking in the oven is heavenly and for some people will bring back good memories to boot. In this crazy and uncertain time, having some treats and comfort food can be just the ticket. My husband said he looked forward to the treats I made for him - and he enjoyed them with whatever sense of smell or taste he could still muster up. So go ahead and have the brownie! And enjoy every bite!

See the recipe section for a yummy brownie recipe that will raise your spirits, pack on a few extra calories and is delicious!

Chapter 20

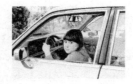

Favorite Recipes

Here are a few of my favorite smoothies, soups, entrées, and desserts that I created and whipped up for my husband during his cancer ordeal. All the recipes I've included in this chapter are soft, smooth, and tasty without being spicy. And, they are easy for a throat cancer patient to eat. With the exception of high-calorie smoothies, all my recipes can be enjoyed by the caregiver, as well - and served to guests with confidence. By preparing foods that the patient as well as the whole family can eat, you'll cut down on prep and cooking time, which is great!

In general, I cook primarily with organic ingredients, as my husband and I switched to eating healthy, organic and whole grain foods more than 15 years ago. If this is not you, don't worry about changing everything in your life right now. Do what you can and save the biggest lifestyle changes for later. Wholesome, home-cooked foods *(organic or not)* are much healthier than pre-packaged foods that require chemical stabilizers, additives, and preservatives to maintain a long shelf life. Plus, pre-packaged foods often contain high amounts of salt and/or sugar. Check the labels to see for yourself.

Buy the freshest ingredients whenever you can. If you're not eating organic, you can eliminate some pesticide residues by cutting off and discarding the peels from fruits and veggies. Alternatively, consider washing non-organic fruits and veggies with special soap solutions designed to get rid of pesticide residues. Health food stores usually carry them as well as more detailed information about these products.

Don't panic about the price of eating whole foods. After all, you're trying to give your loved one a fighting chance at prolonging their life. This is not the right time to skimp on healthy things. Put it in perspective.

Regarding salt, I use either potassium salt or no salt at all. I also don't add salt to any of my recipes that call for pre-packaged broths or sauces, as these products already have salt in them. If you're a salt-lover, you will probably want to add salt to my recipes.

Since you'll be tracking calories, I've added approximate calories per serving to my recipes. Bear in mind that these really are approximate calories, as brands can vary widely in what their ingredients are and how many calories per serving. Low-fat coconut milk, for instance, is ⅓ the calories of regular coconut milk. Teriyaki sauces can vary from 20 to 40 calories per tablespoon, and ice creams can be all over the map. So be sure to check your food labels to verify calories.

About Smoothies
Smoothies are great. I can't say enough good things about them. For starters, you can pack lots of calories and nutrition into a smoothie and they're easy to eat and digest. Smoothies can also make life easier for the caregiver by keeping everyday ingredients relatively simple and consistent. We bought some things in bulk, like cases of rice milk

and large bags of frozen fruits. Do whatever it takes to streamline things.

You can store the smoothie mixture in a large container in the fridge and serve it in portions throughout the day. This is especially useful for the 1,500 - 2,500 calorie versions. Smoothies can be easily transported and/or reheated. And they taste delicious. We made a fresh batch of smoothie each day during the treatment regime and for a month or two after treatments ended. Thin smoothies with water or juice and be sure to put them through a sieve if administering through a feeding tube. Adjust the ingredients and quantities to your specific needs.

To simplify prep time, buy fresh fruit already cleaned and sliced. For turning nuts into more of a powder, prep them in bulk by buying a pound or more of nuts and grinding them in small batches in a blender or food processor. Be sure to store whole or ground nuts in a sealed container in the fridge until ready to use.

For the smoothie base, feel free to use soymilk, rice milk, cow's milk, goat milk, almond milk, etc. Soy, dairy, and goat milk have the most protein per cup. Using part coconut milk or frozen coconut milk is also a wonderful, nutritious addition.

For adding or substituting fruits, we had great success with seedless watermelon, cantaloupe, and defrosted frozen peaches. Fruits can be up to 1 – 2 cups. Be sure to check the calories on the fruits you want to use, for instance: peaches have more calories than watermelon. And, be sure to sieve out the seeds from strawberries and berries, etc.

A note about coconut oil: Make sure the coconut oil is added after everything is blended. Adding the warmed oil directly on top of ice cream can make the oil harden. An easy way to melt the coconut oil is to put the oil in a small cup or bowl and add a small amount of warm water, mixing until the oil is dissolved.

About protein powders: There are many kinds of protein powders, including soy. We chose a very simple, unadulterated, rice protein powder that didn't have all kinds of extra vitamins, supplements, fillers, or questionable ingredients. Rule of thumb: when you read a label and don't understand the ingredients, do a little research and make sure it's right for you - or just skip it. Life is complicated enough and you don't need to be worried about one more thing.

About Soups
My soups can all be pureed to a velvety smooth consistency or thinned to a liquid suitable for administering through a feeding tube, if necessary. When serving through a feeding tube, be sure to puree the soup through a sieve after blending, and make sure the soup is no hotter than room temperature.

If using a blender to puree the soup, an immersion-style blender works best, as you can puree the soup right in the soup pot. If using a counter top blender for pureeing, remove all the steamed veggies and place in a large bowl before pureeing. Pour some of the cooking liquid *(1-2 cups)* into the blender and add a few cups of the cooked veggies. Puree until smooth. Return pureed mixture to the soup pot and blend the rest of the veggies and liquid in batches until everything is pureed.

Take precautions when blending warm soup in a blender. Do not blend when ingredients are piping hot. Be sure to fill blender no more than half full of veggies and cooking liquid, as warm soup can expand and overflow. Make sure the lid is pressed securely onto the blender - and cover the lid with a kitchen towel. Hold towel securely over top of blender while motor is running. Do not walk away from the blender while it is running and be careful not to burn yourself! See your blender manual for safety tips.

Except for the chicken soup recipe, most soups are pretty low in calories and are not meant to be the main course for the patient unless you add more protein and fat before serving. You can bump up calories in soups by adding ingredients to each serving, such as: a few ounces of cooked meats, fish, or tofu; a tablespoon of sesame or olive oil; a dollop of sour cream, yogurt, or a sprinkle of cheese, etc.

In general, I find it much easier to cook lots of veggies if I've already prepped, cleaned, and chopped all or most of my ingredients ahead of time. That way, I can just dump the ingredients into the sauté pans or soup pots and away we go. If you have to cook when you're tired or rushed, it will simplify things for you to have things ready in advance. When you have a little time *(ha ha - when's that?)*, just chop up some extra veggies and put them in bags in the fridge or freezer. You'll thank yourself later.

About Entrées
I've included some of our favorite entrée recipes that are smooth, liquid, soft, or have plenty of sauce. This makes them easier for the patient to eat. They also smell delicious, which is a big plus. The loaf

recipes are especially great for cooking in quantity and freezing some for later. While they require substantial prep time, these recipes will cut down on cooking and prep time down the road *(hooray for microwaves!)*.

About Desserts
The desserts I've included in this chapter are yummy and can add anywhere from 200 to 500 extra calories in one go. This is great, especially at the end of the day when extra calories may be needed. And yes - you can puree any of my desserts and put them through a feeding tube, if needed. Just be sure to have the patient get a good whiff of what they'll be eating so they know what a treat it is!

For caregivers, if you're watching your weight, leave off the whipped cream or ice cream, or cut your portion in half. But remember to savor every delicious morsel free of guilt trips or regrets. Life is precious. Enjoy every moment!

For suggestions on specific brands of ingredients we like, check the Resources chapter.

Smoothies

Caregiver's Smoothie
(approximately 400 calories total)

1 cup unsweetened soymilk
1 large banana
½ cup watermelon
½ cup cantaloupe
1 Tbsp. lecithin granules
1 Tbsp. ground flax seeds
1 Tbsp. rice protein powder

Blend the soymilk, banana, watermelon, and cantaloupe. Add lecithin granules, ground flax seeds, and protein powder. Blend until smooth and creamy. Enjoy!

Note:
While I had smoothie ingredients out for my husband, I would often make a nutritious but lower-calorie smoothie for myself first. When you've already got all the ingredients out for the patient, you might as well take care of yourself, too!

Banana-peach Smoothie with Coconut
(approximately 1,550 calories total)

2 cups unsweetened soymilk
1 large banana
¼ cup ground walnuts
1 Tbsp. lecithin granules
1 Tbsp. ground flax seeds
1 cup *"Coconut Bliss"* frozen dessert or vanilla ice cream
7 ozs. frozen peach slices, defrosted
2 Tbsp. coconut oil, warmed to a liquid consistency
2 Tbsp. rice protein powder

In a blender, combine the rice milk, bananas, ground walnuts, ground flax seeds, and lecithin granules. Soften the ice cream/frozen dessert and blend into the smoothie mixture along with fresh strawberries or your choice of fruits. Pour in the warmed coconut oil followed by the rice protein and blend until smooth and creamy. Enjoy!

Strawberry-banana Coconut Smoothie
(approximately 1,500 calories total)

2 cups rice milk
1 large banana
¼ cup ground walnuts
1 Tbsp. lecithin granules
1 Tbsp. ground flax seeds
1 cup *"Coconut Bliss"* frozen dessert or vanilla ice cream
½ cup fresh strawberries
2 Tbsp. coconut oil, warmed to a liquid consistency
2 Tbsp. rice protein powder

In a blender, combine the rice milk, bananas, ground walnuts, ground flax seeds, and lecithin granules. Soften the ice cream/frozen dessert and blend into the smoothie mixture along with fresh strawberries or your choice of fruits. Pour in the warmed coconut oil followed by the rice protein and blend until smooth and creamy. Enjoy!

John's Favorite Ultra Smoothie

(approximately 2,500 calories total)

2 cups rice milk

2 bananas

½ cup ground walnuts

2 Tbsp. lecithin granules

2 Tbsp. ground flax seeds

2 cups *"Coconut Bliss"* frozen dessert or vanilla ice cream

1 cup fresh strawberries

3 Tbsp. coconut oil, warmed to a liquid consistency

4 Tbsp. rice protein powder

In a blender, combine the rice milk, bananas, ground walnuts, ground flax seeds, and lecithin granules. Soften the ice cream/frozen dessert and blend into the smoothie mixture along with fresh strawberries or your choice of fruits. Pour in the warmed coconut oil followed by the rice protein and blend until smooth and creamy. Enjoy!

Note:
I created this smoothie recipe so my husband could easily consume 2,500 calories without much trouble. We would typically store the smoothie in a large container in the fridge, and portion it out throughout the day. It makes 5 - 6 cups and tastes delicious.

Soups

Carrot-ginger Soup
Makes 6 servings @ approximately 160 calories each

5 cups peeled and diced carrots
2 cups chopped sweet or red onions *(1 medium onion)*
2 cups peeled and diced yams or sweet potatoes *(1 medium yam)*
1 Tbsp. peeled and grated fresh ginger
1 ½ cups unsweetened soymilk
4 cups chicken stock

Place all ingredients in a soup pot and cover with a lid. Bring to a boil, then lower temperature to medium heat. Cook soup for at least 30 minutes, making sure all vegetables are cooked until soft. Cool for five to ten minutes.

Blend soup until creamy and smooth. You can blend either in small batches in a blender - or with a hand-held immersion blender right in the soup pot. Eat as is or top with fresh, chopped chives and a dollop of sour cream or plain yogurt. Enjoy!

Note:
This is a simple, nourishing, and yummy soup! For best results, use the freshest, tastiest carrots available. Our favorite carrots that make the most delicious soup are the heirloom "rainbow" carrots that come in bunches of deep red, yellow, and orange. Try it!

Broccoli-Shitake Soup

Makes 8 servings
approximately 100 calories each for vegetarian version & approximately
330 calories each with chicken and Parmesan

5 cups chopped broccoli *(one large head)*
2 cups sliced shitake mushrooms
2 cups chopped sweet or red onions
1 jar artichoke hearts, chopped *(14 oz.)*
2 cups unsweetened soymilk
4 cups mushroom or chicken stock

Optional:
1 ½ lbs. diced boneless, skinless chicken thighs
2 Tbsp. olive or canola oil
Sage, thyme, oregano, dried chives, salt
Grated Parmesan or Pecorino cheese

Place broccoli, mushrooms, onions, artichoke hearts, soymilk, and stock in a soup pot and cover with a lid. Bring to a boil, then lower temperature to a simmer. Simmer soup for at least 30 minutes, making sure all vegetables are cooked until soft. Cool for five to ten minutes.

Blend soup until creamy and smooth. You can blend either in small batches in a blender - or with a hand-held immersion blender right in the soup pot.

If adding chicken: while soup is cooking, place oil in a large fry pan on medium heat. Add diced chicken and sprinkle lightly with sage, thyme, oregano, dried chives, and a little salt. Stir and continue sautéing chicken until cooked through *(6-8 minutes)*. Adjust seasonings to taste.

For the caregiver and/or family, ladle soup into serving dishes and top with sautéed chicken and two tablespoons of Parmesan cheese. For the patient, be sure to puree the chicken into the vegetarian soup. Make it smooth and creamy. Enjoy!

Susan's Famous "Green Soup"

Makes 8 servings @ approximately 100 calories each

2 cups peeled and diced yams or sweet potatoes (*1 medium*)
2 cups peeled and diced carrots
2 cups diced broccoli
2 cups diced cauliflower
2 cups diced zucchini
1 cup sliced shitake mushrooms
1 ½ cups fresh spinach leaves
¼ cup chopped, fresh parsley
½ cup finely chopped red or sweet onions
3 medium garlic cloves, chopped

Optional ingredients:
¼ cup fresh basil or cilantro
1 tsp. peeled and chopped fresh ginger

This soup is made by layering the veggies in a large soup pot and steaming them until tender. Then blending everything into a pureed soup. It is simple to prep and can easily be frozen in small servings (*2-4 servings per container*). Here's what to do:

Place a steaming basket in a large soup pot and fill with water up to the bottom of the steaming basket. Layer the veggies evenly from the bottom up in the following order: directly on the steamer place the diced yams; then a layer of carrots; a layer of broccoli and cauliflower; a layer of zucchini; a layer of mushrooms. The top layer

119

is a bed of spinach leaves. On top of the spinach leaves, place the parsley *(and basil or cilantro)*. Then top it off with the onions and garlic *(and ginger)*. Place a lid on the pot and bring the steaming water to a boil. Turn down the heat to medium and continue steaming the veggies until they are soft *(20-30 minutes)*. Remember to check the water occasionally and add more if needed.

Let the steamed veggies cool down for ten minutes or so. Remove the steaming basket and pour the steaming liquid into a bowl or measuring cup. Return the veggies to the soup pot and pour in some of the cooking liquid. With a hand held immersion blender, blend the steamed veggies. Add more cooking liquid, as needed - until you reach the desired consistency. I usually make this soup rather thick, but you can add more water or stock to thin to your preference. Enjoy!

Note:
I love this soup. Whenever I'm feeling punky or in need of a nutritional boost, I whip up a batch of this stuff. I've been making this soup for many years. It's chock full of nutrition, needs very little seasoning, and is quite versatile as a base. It is not an exact science. Use more veggies or less. Mix and match your favorite veggies. If you don't like spinach, cabbage works great. You can also add cooked, steamed beets - but I would steam them separately from the green soup and add them when you blend.
After blending the soup, feel free to add bits of cooked chicken, beef, shrimp, or tofu - which you can also blend into the soup. You can also sprinkle cheese on top of individual servings, which is how I usually like to eat it. A sprinkle of freshly grated Pecorino Romano cheese is my

favorite. I usually do not use spices in this soup, as the natural flavors are really great. A sprinkle of salt on top is all you might need.

Dr. Grant's Healing 'n Hearty Chicken Zoup
Makes 6 - 8 servings
For 6 servings with rice: approximately 430 calories/per serving
For 8 servings with rice: approximately 325 calories/per serving

3 quarts chicken stock
1 lb. chicken thighs or breasts, diced *(1 ¼ lbs.)*
3 Tbsp. olive oil
1 medium onion, finely chopped *(sweet white or red onions)*
3-4 cloves garlic, finely chopped
1 cup diced shitake mushrooms
1 cup diced crimini mushrooms
2-3 large carrots, peeled and diced
1 celery stalk, diced
2 zucchini, diced
1 can Great Northern Beans or Navy Beans - rinsed and strained
1 Bay leaf
A pinch of sage, thyme, oregano, and salt-free seasoning
A few sprinkles of dried chives
1 cup elbow macaroni or small pasta shells *(4 oz.)*
1 cup brown rice
Secret ingredient: a large dollop of pure love

Pour 3 quarts of chicken stock into a large soup pot on medium-high heat and bring to a boil. While the stock is coming up to a boil, warm 2 Tbsp. olive oil in a large fry pan. Sauté the chicken until lightly browned on both sides. You do not need to cook the chicken all the way through at this point, as the chicken will finish cooking in the soup. Remove the chicken from the pan and set aside.

Warm another tablespoon of oil in the pan and add the onions, garlic, mushrooms, carrots, celery, and zucchini. Sauté the veggies until they begin to soften.

Carefully spoon the sautéed veggies and the sautéed chicken into the boiling chicken stock. Add the cooked beans, the bay leaf, and the rest of the seasonings - especially *"the love."* Bring the chicken stock back up to a rolling boil and then turn down to a low boil. Cover soup pot with lid and cook for 1 ½ hrs., adding more chicken stock, as needed. Taste the soup broth and adjust seasonings as needed.

While the soup is cooking, place 1 cup brown rice plus 2 cups water in a medium saucepan. Bring to a boil, then simmer 45 minutes or until soft and fluffy.

During the last 20-25 minutes of cooking the chicken soup, add the pasta. This will make the pasta soft and it will take on the flavors of the soup.

When the soup is finished cooking, let it cool for ten to fifteen minutes. Then, ladle out some of the soup into a blender and puree until smooth. If desired, add a scoop of brown rice and puree it into the blended soup *(this makes it extra thick and creamy)*.

Note:
This soup is a variation on grandma's chicken soup. Like my other soups, you can puree some of it for the patient, and leave some of it intact with all

the chunks and textures for the caregiver. Or, blend the whole thing! It tastes yummy either way.

My chicken soup can also be pureed to a very smooth consistency and thinned to a liquid that can be administered through a feeding tube quite easily. To do this, puree soup in a blender and then strain through a sieve. If serving through a feeding tube, make sure the soup is no hotter than room temperature. If adding rice before pureeing, be sure the rice is blended until smooth and creamy; especially if you are feeding through a tube (rice can get sticky!).

And one more thing: I like to keep extra chicken stock on hand, just in case. This soup can thicken overnight in the fridge, and you may want to thin it out with extra stock or water, as needed.

Entrées

Chicken Teriyaki with a Twist
Makes 6 servings @ approximately 300 calories each
(500 calories if served over 1 cup pasta)

6 boneless, skinless chicken thighs *(1 ¼ lbs.)*
14 oz. artichoke heart, quartered & rinsed *(1 can)*
8 oz. fresh mushrooms - either whole, quartered, or sliced
1 cup gluten-free or regular teriyaki sauce

Preheat the oven to 350 degrees. Pour a thin layer of teriyaki sauce in the bottom of an oblong baking dish *(9"x12")*. Rinse the chicken thighs and make 3 diagonal slices along the tops of each piece of chicken. Place the pieces of chicken, bottom side up - in the baking dish on top of the teriyaki sauce. Surround the chicken pieces with the mushrooms and artichoke hearts, tucking them in here and there. Pour the remaining teriyaki sauce evenly on top of the chicken.

Bake for ½ hr. and remove from oven. Turn the pieces of chicken over and spoon some teriyaki sauce on top of each piece of chicken. Put the dish back in the oven and bake for ½ hour more. Remove from oven and let cool slightly before serving. Can be served over rice or pasta and alongside your favorite steamed vegetables.

Note: We found this dish to be soft and easy to chew, especially with a few extra spoonfuls of teriyaki sauce. My husband was able to eat dishes like this throughout most of his treatment regime and again soon after. It's one of his favorite dishes and if I'm not mistaken, we even pureed it and fed it to him through the feeding tube!

Outrageously Yummy Turkey Meatloaf
Makes 2 loaves!
8 slices per loaf @ approximately 452 calories each
(366 without mozzarella)

I break this recipe into 3 parts: the meat mixture, the sauté mixture, and the liquid mixture. I find it's easier to organize the ingredients this way. Preheat the oven to 350.

In a large mixing bowl add the following:
Ground Turkey *(3 lbs.)*
¾ lb. fresh, mild Italian sausage *(squeeze sausage out of casings & discard casings)*
2 cups rolled oats
2 cups shredded mozzarella
½ cup grated Pecorino Romano or Parmesan cheese

Prep the following for sautéing:
2 red onions, finely chopped
4 cloves of garlic, minced
4 medium carrots, grated
1 ½ cups chopped mushrooms *(crimini, shitake, etc.)*
A handful of chopped parsley *(cut off long stems & discard)*

Create a liquid mixture with the following
(a 4-cup measuring cup works well for this)
3 lightly beaten eggs
½ cup ketchup

2 Tbsp. Dijon mustard
Dash of Worcestershire sauce
Sprinkle in salt, sage, thyme, oregano, garlic powder, & dried chives

Directions

Sauté chopped onions and garlic until soft. Add carrots, mushrooms, and parsley. Cook until soft but not cooked all the way through. Cool this mixture.

Mix all ingredients in large mixing bowl until just evenly mixed. Do not over-mix, as this causes the meatloaf to be tough. Kneading the mixture with your hands works best.

Put meatloaf into 2 greased 9"x5" loaf pans, rounding the mixture on top. Place on a baking sheet to catch the drips. Cook at 350 degrees for 1 ½ to 2 hours - until the loaves reach 170 degrees. Cool on a rack for 15 minutes before serving.

Serve with steamed and mashed potatoes or yams and your favorite steamed veggies. To add some extra calories and additional creaminess, top potatoes with sour cream and butter or a good quality olive oil.

Note:
We love this meatloaf. It is moist and full of flavor. Because it is a soft and moist meatloaf my husband was easily able to eat it. My meatloaf can be eaten cold or warm and will keep well when frozen. I often make one loaf "for now" and cut the other loaf into individual servings that I freeze for later. 16-20 servings are worth the effort!

Carl's Favorite Thai Scallops
Makes 4 servings @ approximately 735 calories/serving
(427 calories/serving with "lite" coconut milk)

2 Tbsp. canola or olive oil
4 cloves of minced garlic
8 oz. shitake mushrooms, trimmed & sliced
2 zucchinis, sliced thin *(½ lb.)*
1 lb. scallops
14 oz. coconut milk *(1 can)*
½ tsp. coriander
2 Tbsp. chopped cilantro
2 Tbsp. chopped chives
1 lime, cut into wedges
½ lb. linguine, spaghetti, or wide rice noodles
fresh, ground pepper *(for guests only)*

Bring 4 quarts of water to a boil and start cooking the pasta. While pasta is cooking, warm the canola oil in a large fry pan over medium heat. Add garlic and mushrooms and cook until the mushrooms are soft and tender. Add zucchini and stir fry until al dente *(3-5 minutes)*. Add coconut milk along with the fresh and dried herbs and simmer.

While coconut mixture is simmering, rinse scallops and place on an oiled baking sheet. Broil scallops for 3 minutes on each side. Remove scallops from baking sheet and add to the veggie coconut milk mixture. Add the chopped cilantro and chives and cook just a few minutes more, heating everything through. Make sure the scallops are white in color and slightly firm. Drain pasta.

Divide pasta into four servings and spoon onto plates. Ladle the scallop, veggie, and coconut milk mixture over the pasta. Guests can sprinkle freshly ground pepper on their servings. If desired, serve this dish with lime wedges and squeeze juice over scallops. Yum!

Note:
I discovered that scallops, mushrooms, and zucchini were very easy for my husband to chew and swallow throughout most of his treatment regime. And, this recipe smells delicious and enticed him to the dinner table. It is also a very mild dish. Make sure you don't overcook the scallops, or they will become rubbery.

Regarding scallops, you can use fresh scallops or defrosted ones. Large scallops will take a little longer to broil than the small ones. In my experience, chemical-free scallops taste the best. If you haven't heard about the chemicals that are often used in preserving scallops, be sure to ask your friendly, local fish market to explain it to you. They can tell you if their scallops were soaked in preservatives or not. In the U.S., this process is usually not mentioned on bags of frozen scallops unless it says "chemical-free." Chemical-free scallops are usually off-white in color and should smell light and fresh. It is my understanding that in Canada it is against the law to use any preservatives on seafood, so if you're in Canada, no need to worry about this.

Desserts

Fudgey Chocolate Chip Brownies
(gluten-free)
Makes 8 servings @ approximately 410 calories each
(without whipped cream or ice cream)

4 ozs. unsweetened organic baking chocolate

8 Tbsp. organic extra-virgin coconut oil

1 ½ cups organic sugar

2 tsp. vanilla extract

4 eggs, beaten

1 cup organic gluten-free flour

½ cup finely chopped or ground walnuts or pecans

½ cup gluten-free, semi-sweet chocolate chips

3 Tbsp. grated, unsweetened coconut

Melt coconut oil and baking chocolate in a double boiler over medium heat. Stir often until thoroughly melted.

Remove melted chocolate from heat and let it cool for 5 minutes. Do not let it harden.

Stir sugar and vanilla into chocolate mixture until blended. Then, blend in eggs; fold in flour; and fold in nuts and chocolate chips.

Grease an 8"x8" baking pan and pour batter evenly into baking pan. Sprinkle grated coconut on top of batter.

Bake at 350 degrees for 30-35 minutes. Serve warm with a scoop of vanilla ice cream or a dollop of whipped cream. Yum!

Note:

This recipe does not need to be made gluten-free. You can certainly use regular baking flour and chocolate chips. If the patient is having difficulty swallowing, make sure you grind the nuts and be sure to finely chop the chocolate chips. This recipe is delicious for both the caregiver and the patient. Win-win!

Coconut Custard
Makes 6 servings @ approximately 188 calories each
(without whipped cream, fruit, etc.)

4 eggs, beaten
1 ½ cups unsweetened soymilk
1 cup coconut milk
⅓ cup maple syrup
Dash of nutmeg
½ tsp. vanilla
½ tsp. cinnamon

Beat eggs. Wiz in the other ingredients and beat until smooth. I prefer to use an electric mixer or a blender. You can also mix by hand.

Pour custard mixture into a baking dish *(8"x8" is perfect)*. Set baking dish into a larger baking dish and fill the outer pan with warm water, almost up to the level of the custard.

Bake custard for 45 minutes at 350 degrees or until firm on top. Carefully remove custard pan from water pan. Cool to room temperature before serving. Great topped with whipped cream and/or warm fruit, such as blueberries. Keep refrigerated.

Note:
This creamy, yummy dessert is easy to make, easy to swallow, and easy to digest. If you don't want to use coconut milk, just use 2 cups regular soymilk and ½ cup unsweetened soymilk total.

Magical Maple Bread Pudding
Makes 8 servings @ approximately 520 calories each

3 Tbsp. softened margarine
1 loaf whole grain or spelt bread, sliced *(approximately 20 oz.)*
1 cup blueberries *(frozen are fine)* - or - 1 cup raisins
4 eggs
4 cups unsweetened soymilk
1 cup maple syrup
2 tsp. vanilla extract
1 tsp. cinnamon
Dash of nutmeg

Preheat oven to 375 degrees. Coat the bottom and sides of a 9"x13" glass baking pan with a few tablespoons of unsalted, soft margarine. Place loaf of bread in baking pan with the slices standing up. Tuck the blueberries or raisins in between the slices. Sprinkle any extra fruit along the sides of the bread.

Beat the four eggs until they're frothy and add in the 4 cups of soymilk, 1 cup of maple syrup, 2 tsp. vanilla, 1 tsp. of cinnamon, and a dash of nutmeg. Beat until smooth.

Pour the liquid over the bread slices and gently press the bread with a spatula to help it absorb the egg mixture. Do this repeatedly every ten to 15 minutes for one hour. The bread will soften and expand, filling the pan.

Bake the bread pudding approximately one hour. Pudding should be puffy and a little brown on top. Let cool slightly. Cut into squares and serve warm. If you can tolerate dairy, add a dollop of whipped cream or vanilla yogurt on top. Or, warm some maple syrup and drizzle on top.

Be sure to refrigerate any leftover pudding, as it will keep for a few days if chilled. Bread pudding tastes best if eaten within a day of cooking. Pudding can be eaten chilled or can be reheated on low heat in the microwave or oven.

Note:
This is one of our favorite bread puddings. The recipe has evolved over the years to be wheat-free and dairy-free. It's a healthier version than the typical white bread, sugar and milk variety. Use a whole grain, seedless bread. If it has a hearty crust, slice off the crusts before adding the bread to the pan. Consider using organic or transitional blueberries or raisins, as their non-organic cousins may be loaded with pesticides.
I wouldn't normally recommend raisins (too chewy) for a throat cancer patient. But since the raisins are soaked in the custard mixture, they plump up and are juicy and easy to eat.

Sautéed Bananas A La Mode
Makes 2 servings @ approximately 240 calories
(or as much as 480 calories with ice cream)

2 large bananas, peeled and sliced lengthwise down the middle
2 Tbsp. margarine or coconut oil
Dash of cinnamon *(optional)*
Ice cream or non-dairy frozen dessert

Melt the margarine or coconut oil in a large fry pan. Place the banana slices in the pan on medium heat and cook 3-4 minutes on each side, or until bananas are slightly browned and soft. Add a dash of cinnamon, if desired.

Remove bananas from pan and place on dessert plates. Add a scoop or two of your favorite frozen dessert or yogurt. Be sure to serve the bananas while they are still warm. Delish!

Note:
As an alternative, you can serve this dessert topped with warm blueberries and whipped cream. For the caregiver, top with chopped pecans, too.

Chapter 21

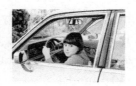

Tools, Supplies, and What to Keep in Your Cupboard

Check out the following tools, equipment, groceries, and supplies listed in this chapter. In our experience, we found these items to be quite helpful - and in some cases, essential to the healing process. See the *Checklists and Shopping lists* chapter for user-friendly shopping guides to use while you're out and about.

Keeping Track of Calories

√ **Calorie counter** - whether it's a softbound reference book, a software program, or an app for your handheld device, do whatever works for you and makes your life easy. We found that simply keeping a calorie counting book handy along with a small notepad for tallying daily amounts was extremely helpful and all that was needed. Whatever method you choose, remember it needs to be something that can be shared between caregiver and patient, especially as the patient becomes more independent.

√ **Food log** - a notebook or pad of paper works just fine. The patient will need to eat many more calories than normal, and it is important to track the calories religiously, or the patient will just keep losing weight. Believe it or not, my husband needed to eat almost 4,000 calories a day just to maintain his weight - and that was after losing over 30 pounds!

√ **Tip** - We found it easier to pack in ½ - ¾ of a day's worth of calories in one smoothie, which was usually 4-6 cups of smoothie at a time *(one blender full)*. See recipe chapter for details.

Tools for the Kitchen

√ **Blender for making smoothies, etc.** - We used a freestanding blender as well as a hand-held immersion blender. You'll need a blender that is more of a *"work horse"* if you're going to make daily smoothies and pureed soups, so make sure to buy a good one. Buying an extra glass carafe for the blender is also a good idea. The freestanding blender is perfect for making smoothies, while the immersion-style blender is great for pureeing hot soups directly into the soup pot. This is much safer than blending soups in a freestanding blender, as hot foods can expand and pop the lid off! Bonus: there'll be fewer utensils to clean if you use an immersion-style blender with soups.

√ **Food scale** - We prefer a relatively flat version that sits on the counter and measures **primarily** ounces *(needed for counting calories)*. Ours is digital, but there are manual ones as well.

√ **Measuring cups** - (needed for counting calories).

√ **Measuring spoons** - Tablespoons, teaspoons, etc.

√ **Paper plates, cups, bowls, etc.** - Make it easy on yourself - or you'll end up washing dishes every night until midnight and then you'll be really cranky. We even used paper bowls for feeding our dogs. Rinse and recycle them when you're done and you won't feel so guilty about using paper. Just tell yourself you're having lots of picnics!

√ **Storage containers** - Quart, pint, gallon, etc. You'll need quart and pint-sized containers that are good for liquids, such as juices and smoothies - preferably ones you can drink out of, that can pour easily, and are transportable. You'll also need containers for various cut fruit, chopped veggies, etc., as well as the soups you make and possibly freeze. Container options are infinite. My favorites include plastic containers with tightly sealing lids in all shapes and sizes - especially for travel. At home we use tall, glass containers with lids for storing smoothies in the fridge.

√ **Strainers and a Sieve** - I can't tell you enough how helpful these gadgets are. The sieve we purchased is an old-fashioned sieve - which is basically a large, mesh food strainer with a crank. While blending and pureeing is great, sieving will help remove little seeds from fruit *(especially berries like strawberries)* or the extra bits a blender can't completely puree. Sieving eliminates the problem patients can have with choking and coughing on little bits of food that get stuck in the throat. Sieving is also perfect for getting the right consistency to put through the feeding tube. *(Thanks to Lucysrealfood.com for the sieve idea, which was a godsend.)*

141

Grocery items to have on hand

- **Aloe juice.** Buy preservative-free, if at all possible.

- **Applesauce** in jars or in individual servings. Homemade is great, too.

- **Avocados.** Easy to make creamy and smooth and wonderful for adding some extra calories and nutrients.

- **Broths,** such as chicken or mushroom. We used these for soup bases as well as for making thinner consistencies to soups, etc. Look for low sodium versions of broths, as salt content per serving can be high.

- **Coconut milk** - full fat or low fat.

- **Dairy** *(if not sensitive to this)*: yogurt, sour cream, really good ice cream *(no artificial colorings, flavorings, or preservatives)*. My husband's favorite ice cream is Haagen-Dazs, which has only 5 simple ingredients and packs in a lot of calories, i.e., 1 pint is 1,000 calories.

- **Flax Seeds.** Flax seeds are a wonderful addition to smoothies, as they are high in Omega-3 fatty acids. Buy them already ground or if you're buying the seeds, be sure to grind them as finely as possible before adding to smoothies, etc.

- **Fresh fruits**, especially bananas. And if available: watermelon, cantaloupe, peaches, strawberries, etc. Acidity is a problem for throat cancer patients, so avoid using oranges, pineapples, and lemons.

- **Fresh veggies** for pureeing: zucchini, carrots, yams, broccoli, beets, etc. Frozen peas are a great addition, too. Greens are also great .(*See recipe chapter for wonderful soup ideas.*)

- **Frozen coconut ice cream,** such as Coconut Bliss (*my hubbie's favorite*). Bliss uses agave for a sweetener, which is low on the glycemic index and is easy for the body to utilize. It doesn't spike one's blood sugar, and this is a good thing! Alternative frozen desserts made of soymilk, rice milk, etc. - are great for people who are allergic or sensitive to dairy.

- **Frozen fruits:** peaches, cherries, blueberries, and strawberries. Just remember: berry seeds will need to be sieved out of the smoothies before serving.

- **Fruit juices:** apple, peach, apricot, mango, etc. Avoid the acidic ones, such as orange, grapefruit, tomato, etc. Acidic juices can literally be quite painful to drink or swallow. My husband enjoyed drinking grape juice during the first couple of weeks, but then found it to be too acidic after that. We found nectars to be easier to swallow. Nectars also seemed to coat the throat, which my husband experienced as quite soothing.

- **Lecithin** (*granulated*).

- **Liquid vitamins:** you can even put these through the feeding tube, which is great.

- **Nuts:** walnuts, almonds.

- **Oils:** olive, sesame, canola, and coconut oils. Coconut oil hardens at room temperature, so be sure to gently melt it before using. I like to warm a few tablespoons in a cup in the microwave for 20 seconds or so before adding to smoothies.

- **Proteins:** Fresh fish, chicken, tofu, eggs, and beans.

- **Protein powder.** We use a very simple one that is made of rice protein.

- **Soymilk, rice milk, and/or almond milk.** In our case, we did not want to overdo it on the dairy, as dairy can increase inflammation and congestion, which my husband had a devil of a time dealing with. *(Per my nutritionist and the naturopaths I've worked with, limiting or eliminating dairy can be very beneficial for decreasing inflammation and congestion.)*

- **Spirulina** *(powdered)*. Add a teaspoon to smoothies for extra nutritional benefits.

- **Sweeteners:** honey, agave syrup, and maple syrup.

For First Aid *(these are all over-the-counter/non-prescription)*
- Aquaphor *(for moisturizing and protecting the skin)*.

- Aloe Vera gel *(as pure as possible)*.

- Bandage tape - hurt-free paper tape, if possible. Available in a dispenser.

- Biotene gum, toothpaste, and mouthwash. *(Recommended by our dentist, Biotene temporarily helps alleviate the symptoms of dry mouth.)*

- Disposable vinyl or latex gloves by the box *(make sure you aren't allergic to these)*.

- Domeboro *(a drying agent for the radiated skin, if needed)* - and a container to mix it in. Only purchase and use if your doctor recommends it.

- Facial tissue by the box & travel-sized ones, too.

- Gauze pads: 2"x2" or larger.

- Hydrogen peroxide.

- Lip balm.

- Lozenges- to help stimulate salivary glands and soothe the throat.

- Nasal Saline and/or Netti pot - helped reduce sinus inflammation and clear sinuses.

- Olbas (*natural, eucalyptus-based inhalant for nasal congestion*).

- Oral Thermometer.

- Rubbing alcohol.

- Salt for salt-water rinses and gargling. Ratio: ½ teaspoon per 8 oz. cold or room temperature water.

- Scissors for cutting gauze & tapes.

- Small garbage bags (*for disposing of medical waste*).

- Sterile gauze rolls.

- Telfa pads (*or non-stick pads*): 4" or larger.

- Tongue depressors for spreading Aquafor, antibiotic or other creams onto Telfa pads.

- Tri-Salts (*by Ecological Formulas*) - is a powder that you dissolve in a glass of water. We find it to be highly effective as an alkalanizer, which really helps relieve acid indigestion.

- Un-petroleum jelly (*petroleum jelly without the petroleum :=*)

- Vitamin E oil or capsules (*we mix aloe gel with the vitamin E*).

- Washcloths and towels.

To-Go Bag
- Aloe Vera gel.

- Bandages, salves, & tape, if needed.

- Biotene gum.

- Bottled Water.

- Clothes: extra shirt, t-shirt, bandana. If it's summer, be sure to bring a sun hat, as the cancer treatments and medications can cause sun-sensitivity.

- Facial tissue.

- Juice *(non-acidic, such as apple, pear, or peach)*.

- Lip Balm.

- Meals & snacks - especially whatever your loved one can easily absorb to keep their calories up *(smoothies, pureed soups, desserts, etc.)*.

- Medications the patient is currently taking.

- Nasal saline such as *Ocean.*

- Something to read or do. During the first few weeks of treatment, my husband was able to do work on his laptop computer during chemo.

- Vitamin E oil.

To Wear

- **Hats** for keeping the sun off the face and neck.

- **Hospital gowns** are very good to have on hand. Hospital-style gowns make it easier for the caregiver to apply creams, salves, and bandages to the patient's neck area or to help access the feeding tube. We asked our health care provider to loan us a couple of gowns during the treatment process and they said, "Yes." See if your clinic will do that for you, too.

- **Kerchiefs, bandanas, and/or scarves.** Why? As the neck gets radiated, it gets red and sensitive, as if it has intense sunburn. The skin can also become extremely sun-sensitive, and needs more protection. Additionally, chafing can be a problem. Kerchiefs, bandanas, and scarves that are soft and lightweight are great for protecting the radiated neck from the elements as well as for privacy for the patient *(their necks can look pretty strange at times!).* The patient's skin also needs to stay hydrated or it will get dry and very tight *(skin can even crack if it's too dry)*, which is quite painful. Bandages may be needed to hold in the salves and ointments on the neck. These can be bulky for the patient and disquieting for others to see. To accommodate bandages, scarves and bandanas need to be somewhat loose or adjustable.

- **Loosely fitting black or dark shirts** and t-shirts were very helpful in hiding the feeding tube, especially when going out in public.

- **Tops that fit loosely around the neck.** Think *"Flash Dance"(80's style workout wear).* Scoop necks and v-necks that are relatively loose - or collars and sweatshirts where the neckline is cut extra wide. We actually snipped open some necklines to make them more comfortable with less chafing. Turtlenecks, if loose, might work in the beginning - and later on after treatment, but during treatment, anything that rubs on the neck can be quite painful.

A note about weight and clothing: Don't be surprised if the patient drops a size or two. During his cancer treatments, my husband dropped 2 sizes in jeans and went from a large to a medium in shirts. So you just might need to go clothes shopping during this ordeal.

Chapter 22

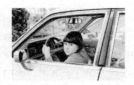

Staying Sane
and Reducing Stress

When thinking about your life right now, are you asking yourself, *"Who wrote this script and why hasn't he/she been fired yet?"* Good. You're on the right chapter! There have been so many times in my life where I wanted to *"fire my scriptwriters"* - especially during times when I couldn't believe what was happening to me or why. The *"My Husband Has Throat Cancer"* chapter was definitely one of them, until I found several silver linings, a lot to be grateful for, and a big reservoir of humor.

I do know this: if you can manage to step back from the inevitable pain, suffering, and daily drama that cancer brings into your life, you just might be able to see the blessings, the life lessons, and even the humor in your situation. I did all three when my husband was ill, and it really helped! Here are some suggestions:

Try reducing or eliminating everyday sources of negativity and stress as much as you can. Here are few simple ways that I find helpful:

- Turn off the news. Most news programs are full of murder, mayhem, and stories of what's wrong with the world. Do you really need to see or hear this right now? I doubt it. Just check your heart rate when you're watching or listening to those stories and you'll see what I mean.

- Ditto for TV shows that are full of violence, brutality, and cruelty. If you have a favorite non-violent show, try recording it to watch later. Skip the commercials filled with violent or shocking movie previews. Skip the junk food commercials. And most of all, skip the drug commercials, especially the ones that focus on pain, suffering, depression, and the wacky side effects the narrators say with their sing-song-y voices. You don't need anything else to worry about right now.

- Update your computer's home page to display something cheerful, uplifting, or altogether neutral. If your home page opens to the news, change it.

- Set limits on your time when dealing with needy or difficult people, even if they are treasured family members, friends, or colleagues. Practice saying "no."

- Resist the temptation to defend your decisions and choices to family, friends, and co-workers. It's exhausting to do this, and most people won't be swayed in their opinions anyway.

- Create a drama-free zone by staying away from people and places that drain you. You'll need all your vital energy and then some to get through this crazy cancer process.

- Give your mind a break from negative thinking. Whenever you notice yourself having painful, negative, or worrisome thoughts, stop them in their tracks. You can do this by visualizing a stop sign and think the word *"Stop!"* Alternatively, you can think to yourself *"Shhhhhhh!"* when troubling thoughts appear, as if someone is asking you to be quiet. I have found both methods work very well. Over time, you can literally retrain your brain to stop thinking negatively.

- Most of all, try to notice and identify the things that add stress to your daily life and do what you can to reduce or eliminate these daily stressors. You may have more control over this than you think!

Add in some positive actions and behaviors to help change your state of mind. Here are a few things that I have found helpful:

- Have a good laugh every day. Laughter is great medicine, so enjoy as much laughter as possible. Because my husband loves jokes, we asked people to email him jokes or send him joke books. He loved it! John began each day by reading jokes and laughing - and of course, memorizing the good jokes to tell again. My husband loves making people laugh, so this was great for everyone!

- Add a little art into your life. Whether it's going to an art museum or local gallery, listening to great music at home or out at a concert, listening to or reading poetry, etc. - art will greatly improve your state of mind. In the movie *"Tune in Tomorrow,"* the lead character says one of my favorite lines: *"When it's raining s**t, the best umbrella you can have is art."* I agree!

- Get out to where there is fresh air and trees and take a walk. You don't have to power-walk or run a marathon. Just go out and get a little *"nature juice"* if you can. If you live in a city, find a lovely park, a beautiful garden, or fountain to visit.

- Take a few minutes each day to do some relaxation exercises such as Qigong or yoga. We found a wonderful Qigong DVD that is 20 minutes long and very relaxing *(see resources)*.

- Close your eyes and do some deep breathing whenever you feel stressed. Inhale and feel your belly fill with air like a big balloon. Exhale and gently squeeze the air out of your belly and organs. Say *"Haaaaahhh"* out loud as you exhale. Repeat several times.

- Journal about your feelings and experiences whenever you feel the need to *"get things out."* Journaling can help relieve anxiety and might also help you get clear about what's going on. Seeing things more clearly may give you the boost you need to help solve your problems.

- If you have a dog that is social and loves people, ask the clinic if you can bring them to the waiting room. At one of the oncology clinics, I was allowed to bring my two little dogs. They were not only a comfort to me and my husband, they also cheered up all the folks in the waiting room. Even the staff looked forward to seeing my *"girls."* It was great!

- Watch funny movies - especially ones that will make you laugh.

- Watch movies that have a happy ending. Don't underestimate the power of *"feeling good"* when you watch people live happily ever after.

- Read uplifting and inspiring books, articles, etc. - especially before bed or upon awakening.

- Most of all, make a list of the things you like to do that make you happy. And make sure you incorporate them into your daily life.

Try to find the silver lining in your situation by asking yourself positive questions. This can be especially helpful when life is difficult, confusing, or painful. The following questions can help shift your thinking away from *"what's wrong"* and into *"what's right."*

- If there was a gift in this experience, what would it be?
- What am I glad I know now that I didn't know before?
- Where in my life do I feel lucky or blessed?
- What people, places, experiences, etc., am I grateful for?
- What steps can I take to actively improve my situation?

The bottom line to staying sane and reducing stress is to do whatever you can to create and sustain a positive environment and state of mind. It may sound a bit simplistic, but *"Out with the bad and in with the good"* can work wonders!

Chapter 23

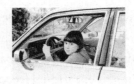

Seeing the Humor

If you're open to seeing the humor in your situation, this chapter is for you. Being able to laugh at or poke fun at yourself may not be your shtick, but it can be a great tool - especially when your drama has reached a crescendo. If you can get yourself to the point where you can see how ridiculous this whole situation is, you just might feel a heck of a lot better.

When life gets tough, I make comedy. I've always been that way. At my house, whenever life gets crazy and we start feeling really spun out of control, one of us will undoubtedly say, *"Is it comedy yet?"* It's a gentle reminder that if we're too caught up in whatever drama has come our way - or - if we're too emotionally charged about a situation or problem, it's bound to get even crazier if we don't take a moment to step back and somehow see the humor. For us, there's always a little humor to be found somewhere. And usually, we don't have to dig too deep to find it.

Sometimes my husband and I will get inspired to sit down and brainstorm some goofy ideas for a product, service, or even lyrics to a song that elevates our crazy situation to humor. After we do this, we usually feel much better afterward, even if it's only for a few moments or a few hours. John and I find that humor will make our attachment to a problem dissipate, which can be quite healing and energizing, as well. As we make sense - or nonsense - out of our difficulties, we've found that fear and emotional suffering can be replaced by joy, contentment, and a feeling of emotional freedom. Of course, making nonsense is the big key here!

To see the humor in your situation, try adding a little comedy right now by doing any of the following:

1. Ask yourself this: If my life is a comedy and not a tragedy, what elements, moments, characters, etc., could I find funny? Where is the humor in this situation?

2. Try seeing the funny side of your situation by making up a goofy song. Take a simple, familiar tune and plug in lyrics about your life. Ham it up and make fun of your situation. Make yourself laugh!

3. As you talk about your problems, imagine you've just inhaled helium and are saying the same words. Hey - maybe you should get a few helium balloons and try this. I doubt you'll be able to stay in a serious or depressed mood.

4. Try naming your cancer situation. Instead of calling it *cancer*, maybe call it Bob or Luella. Naming it helps to put it *"out there"* instead of *"in here."* And, it just might make you laugh!

5. Does your situation remind you of something funny? See what you can come up with. I told my husband he looked *"All puffed out like an Amazonian frog."* Thereafter, he would come up to me saying *"Ribbitt Ribbitt... "* Yes - it was funny! What will tickle *your* funny bone?

6. Take a difficult scenario you're dealing with and write about it in a humorous way. Find the craziness and make it funny. You can give your experiences a little tweak or a noogie and

see how it shifts your frame of mind. My husband called his radiation treatments, *"The $150,000 Radiation Facelift."* I renamed his Lorazapan pills *"Marzipan Pills."* When he was at his very worst, I sat down and wrote some things about his situation that made him laugh out loud. Here's an excerpt:

You wake up and look in the mirror and don't recognize yourself. Suddenly you consider a new career in horror films. The skin on your throat is quite literally the color of a beet, and is oozing yellow ooky stuff. You can't believe it. No one told you this would happen. You try to turn your neck, but it's too stiff because the skin is tight as a drum. Now you think, "Hey - I could play Frankenstein. All I need are those two knobby things sticking out of the sides of my neck and I'm good to go." You go online and look in the LA yellow pages under "agents." Being able to pay your medical bills now looks promising!

You stick out your tongue and say "ahhh" to yourself in the mirror. Wow! Instead of a nice pink tongue, yours looks all mashed up, with more yellow gooky stuff oozing out of the top and sides of your tongue. Now you're inspired to create a new and innovative product line: cancer victim costumes for Halloween. You seriously consider this. After all, you've barely been able to work for the last three months and counting, and you've recently been told by your medical team, "It's going to get worse before it gets better. "

OK - so now you're wondering, "What else has to get worse before I can get better? Will my head fall off and my wife will adeptly and lovingly stitch it back on so I can watch a little comedy?"

You apply the prescribed analgesic cream to your neck. Even the lightest touch sends your eyes rolling back in your head. You grip the sink and wince in between dabs of the ointment. Now you envision yourself in an old Western movie. You're the hero and you've been shot pretty bad. The doc gives you a swig of whiskey but it's not enough to ease the pain. As he digs into your skin to pull the bullet out, you bite down hard on a stick, and think to yourself, "M-O-M-M-Y." You want to scream "M-O-M-M-Y!", but you don't want to scare the neighbors!

So, the bottom line is this: do what you can to gain a humorous perspective about your situation. Your problems, pain, and suffering may not last forever, but your humorous attitude can help get you through the worst of it - and maybe even help others, as well!

Chapter 24

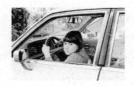

Checklists and Shopping Lists

This chapter contains suggested checklists and shopping lists of items included in the *Tools and Supplies, Getting the Best Nutrition, and Home Remedies* chapters. I find that having checklists are a great help, especially when shopping. Add or subtract items as needed for your own situation. And, make sure the patient is not allergic to anything on your list. For explanations on why these items worked for us, read the related chapters in this book.

A brief note about grocery items: Try buying organic and transitional produce if you can. And, avoid added chemicals and preservatives whenever possible. You don't have to be a food fanatic. Obviously the healthier, fresher, and more high quality the food is, the better it is for the patient - and you!

Tools and supplies before treatment begins
- ○ Blender *(and extra glass carafe)*
- ○ Calorie counter
- ○ Food scale
- ○ Food storage containers with lids
- ○ Large soup pot

o   Measuring cups (*and extras*)
o   Measuring spoons
o   Paper plates, cups, and bowls
o   Pureeing sieve and strainers

Fresh fruits, vegetables, and bulk foods (*reminder: avoid citrus, acidic or spicy foods*)

o   Almonds
o   Avocados
o   Bananas
o   Beets
o   Blueberries
o   Broccoli
o   Brown rice
o   Cantaloupe
o   Carrots
o   Cauliflower
o   Celery
o   Cherries
o   Cilantro
o   Garlic
o   Ginger root
o   Mushrooms - Crimini and Shitake
o   Onions
o   Parsley
o   Peaches
o   Pecans
o   Potatoes
o   Quinoa or other alternative whole grains

- o Raisins
- o Rolled oats
- o Spinach & other steaming greens
- o Strawberries
- o Walnuts
- o Watermelon
- o Yams or sweet potatoes
- o Zucchini

Spices & Seasonings: (*reminder: use spices in moderation*)
- o Bay leaf
- o Black pepper
- o Cinnamon
- o Coriander
- o Dried chives
- o Nutmeg
- o Oregano
- o Sage
- o Salt or potassium salt
- o Salt-free seasoning (*e.g., Vegit*)
- o Thyme
- o Vanilla extract

Dairy: (*reminder: avoid products with hormones & additives*)
- o Milk
- o Sour Cream
- o Yogurt

Oils:
- Coconut oil
- Canola oil
- Olive oil
- Sesame oil

Frozen Fruits & other items:
- Blueberries
- Cherries
- Ice cream or alternative frozen dessert *(e.g., Coconut Bliss)*
- Peaches
- Peas
- Strawberries

Protein: *(reminder: avoid deli meats with nitrates & nitrates)*
- Chicken breasts or thighs *(boneless, skinless)*
- Eggs
- Grated Parmesan or Pecorino Romano cheese
- Ground turkey *(lean)*
- Mild Italian sausage
- Mozzarella or other favorite cheeses
- Salmon
- Scallops
- Tofu
- Turkey breast

Canned or packaged foods: *(reminder: avoid added chemicals and preservatives)*
- Applesauce

- o Artichoke hearts
- o Chicken and/or vegetable broths (*low sodium*)
- o Chocolate chips
- o Coconut milk
- o Dijon mustard
- o Fruit juices & nectars: apple, peach, apricot, and/or mango
- o Grated, unsweetened coconut
- o Great northern beans or navy beans
- o Ketchup
- o Pastas
- o Rolled oats
- o Soymilk, rice milk, or almond milk
- o Sweeteners: honey, maple syrup, white sugar, brown sugar
- o Teriyaki sauce
- o Unsweetened baking chocolate
- o Whole grain bread (*seed-free*)
- o Whole grain flour
- o Worcestershire sauce

Nutritional supplements & vitamins:
- o Aloe Vera juice
- o Digestive enzymes
- o Flax seed (*ground or whole*)
- o Granulated lecithin
- o Liquid calcium/magnesium
- o Protein powder
- o Throat lozenges
- o Tri-Salts

First Aid:

- o   Aloe Vera gel
- o   Aquaphor
- o   Biotene gum and toothpaste
- o   Gauze pads - 2"x2" and larger
- o   Gauze wrap *(by the roll)*
- o   Hurt-free tape
- o   Hydrogen peroxide
- o   Lip Balm
- o   Nasal saline
- o   Olbas
- o   Oral thermometer
- o   Rubbing alcohol
- o   Salt
- o   Scissors for cutting gauze
- o   Telfa pads - 4" or larger
- o   Un-petroleum jelly
- o   Vinyl or latex disposable gloves
- o   Vitamin E oil

To wear:

- o   Hospital gowns
- o   Kerchiefs, bandanas, and/or scarves
- o   Loosely fitting shirts
- o   Scoop or v-neck t-shirts and sweatshirts *(especially black or dark colors)*
- o   Sun hat with visor

Other:

- Facial tissue - boxes & travel-sized
- Funny movies!
- Joke books or other fun things to read
- Small bottles of drinking water (*e.g., spring water*)
- Small garbage bags for medical waste
- Sunscreen

Chapter 25

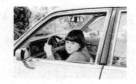

Celebrate - Throw a Party!

O.K. So enough about the fear and uncertainty about what's coming down the pike. Before your loved one starts chemo, radiation, or goes in for surgery, be sure to have a pre-celebration. That's right - celebrate the success of the upcoming ordeal before you begin the process.

My husband's birthday was going to land right about the time he was scheduled to finish his chemo and radiation. And, I figured he wouldn't be able to enjoy eating birthday cake at that point - or maybe not even feel like visiting people then. So I decided to give him an early birthday party before he began his treatments. It was great! I invited a dozen or so of his favorite people and had a wonderful dinner party, complete with a delicious birthday cake. Everyone showed up to hug him, wish him well, and offer their support. It also gave my husband an opportunity to thank people and let them know what they meant to him - and it started John off on his cancer treatment journey a couple of days later with a positive spirit, feeling very loved and taken care of by those around him.

It doesn't need to be anyone's birthday to have a cake, candles, and good wishes. You can buy a cake, make a cake, or have a friend bring one by. Cupcakes are great, too. Blowing out candles and being surrounded by good friends and family is a great morale booster.

So, before treatments begin, have a pre-celebration party, gathering, or just a special dinner for two. This just might be *"what the doctor ordered"* to start you on your journey in a positive way. Try it!

Chapter 26

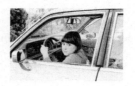

Resources

Information and Assistance

Creating a website for keeping people informed:

www.CaringBridge.org

Feeding tube advice and nutritious recipes for the tube:

www.LucysRealFood.com

Financial help:

www.Cancer.org (*American Cancer Society*)

www.CancerCare.org

www.PatientAdvocate.org

Call your local United Way for programs that can help you

Information and support:

www.CancerCare.org

www.Cancer.org

www.CancerSupportCommunity.org

www.HeadandNeck.org (*Head and Neck Cancer Alliance*)

www.OncoLink.org

www.OralCancerFoundation.org

www.SPONHC (*Support for People with Head and Neck Cancer*)

www.ThroatCancerHelp.com

A Caregiver's Guide To Throat Cancer

In-home nursing:
Ask for lists of local providers from your doctor and/or insurance company

Support for caregivers:
www.LotsaHelpingHands.com
www.nfcacares.org (*The National Family Caregivers Association*)

Ask at your oncology clinic for a list of local support groups for caregivers. If there isn't one in your area, start one!

Nutritional Supplies & Supplements

Note: Products we recommend are those we have used and have found to be helpful. Do your homework and learn more to be sure these products are right for your particular situation. None of the companies listed below solicited us to recommend their products, nor were we paid for any endorsements.

Aloe Vera Juice *(look for preservative-free)*:
George's (*tastes the best!*): www.GeorgesAloe.com
Lily of the Desert Preservative-free Aloe Vera Juice:
www.LilyoftheDesert.com

Calcium/Magnesium *(liquid formula)*:
Bluebonnet Liquid Calcium Magnesium Citrate Plus Vitamin D3:
www.BlueBonnetNutrition.com

Coconut Oil *(extra virgin coconut oil has the most nutrients)*:
Nature's Way Pure Extra Virgin Coconut Oil: www.Naturesway.com
Nutiva Organic Extra Virgin Coconut Oil: www.Nutiva.com
Spectrum: www.SpectrumOrganics.com

Coconut Milk:
Thai Kitchen: www.ThaiKitchen.com

Coconut Dessert: *(frozen)*
Coconut Bliss: www.CoconutBliss.com
Purely Decadent: www.Turtlemountain.com

Digestive Enzymes: *(these are all vegetarian formulas)*
Enzymedica Digest: www.Enzymedica.com
Rainbow Light Advanced Enzyme System: www.RainbowLight.com
Now Plant Enzymes: www.NowFoods.com
Source Naturals: Daily Essential Enzymes: www.SourceNaturals.com

Flax Seeds:
Organic ground premium flaxseed: www.SpectrumOrganics.com

Fruit Juices:
Santa Cruz Organic: www.SantaCruzOrganic.com
Knudsen Juices: www.KnudsenJuices.com

Healthy Oils, such as Olive Oil & Sesame Oil:
www.SprectrumOrganics.com

Immune Boosting Formula:
Wellness Formula - Herbal Resistance by Source Naturals:
www.SourceNaturals.com

Lecithin Capsules:
Barlean's flax oil: www.Barleans.com 800-445-3529

Lecithin Granules:
www.NowFoods.com

Liquid Vitamins:
Nature's Plus Source of Life Liquid Vitamins www.NaturesPlus.com

Orithrush:
Ecological Formulas - (925) 827-2636 (*for oral thrush symptoms*)

Probiotics:
Dr. Ohhira's Probiotics: www.EssentialFormulas.com
PB8: www.NutritionNow.com

Protein Powder:
Nutribiotic Rice Protein (*vanilla*): www.Nutribiotic.com
Lifetime Life's Basics Plant Protein Powder: www.LifetimeVitamins.com

Rice Milk:
Rice Dream: www.TastetheDream.com

Soy Milk: (*carrageenan-free*)
West Soy Organic Original or Unsweetened: www.Westsoy.biz

Tri-Salts:
Ecological Formulas - (925) 827-2636

First Aid Supplies

Topicals:
Aloe Vera Gel: Lily of the Desert Aloe Vera Gelly:
    www.LilyoftheDesert.com

Vitamin E oil: Now E-Oil (*dropper bottle*): www.NowFoods.com
Aquaphor Ointment: www.EucerinUS.com - available at pharmacies
Un-Petroleum Jelly: www.AlbaBotanica.com

Resources

Hurt-free tapes, wraps, and non-stick pads:
Johnson & Johnson: www.jnj.com - available at pharmacies

Other:
Olbas Aromatherapy Inhaler: www.Olbas.com
Biotene products for dry mouth - www.biotene.com - available at pharmacies

Kitchen tools

Blender:
Cuisinart & Kitchen Aid - available at www.Amazon.com

Hand-held immersion-style blender:
Viking Handblender #VHB300PS: www.VikingRange.com

Kitchen scale:
www.SalterHousewares.com (*we use Salter model 1038*)

Sieve/food mill:
Endurance puree sieve by R.S.V.P. International: available at Amazon.com

Exercise DVD's:
For instructional DVD's on exercise and healing: www.Gaiam.com

One of our favorite exercise DVD's:
"Qigong for Stress Relief" with Francesco & Daisy Lee-Garripoli

Afterward

The inspiration for writing this book came from my husband, John Pizzo, who was diagnosed with throat cancer in late March 2010. He underwent intensive chemo and radiation in May/June 2010. At this time (*first quarter of 2012*) John is not entirely symptom-free, but he is cancer-free and living a relatively active, normal, and healthy life. He is glad to be on the other side of cancer, is more appreciative and grateful than ever before, and is looking forward to many more happy years together. We just celebrated our eighteenth year of marriage.

Here is a recent photo I took of John and "the girls" during one of our adventures.

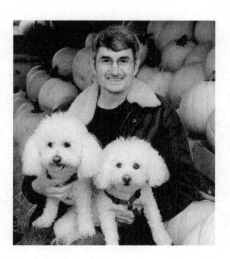

About the Author

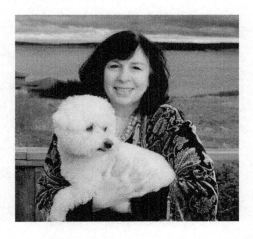

Susan Grant is an artist and writer in the Pacific Northwest who is known for her resourcefulness, can-do attitude, and wonderful sense of humor. Armed with a *Master's Degree in Therapy* and an ongoing education from the *School of Hard Knocks*, Grant shares her wisdom, wit, and life lessons through a series of self-help books. *A Caregiver's Guide to Throat Cancer* is the first of several practical, fun, and informative books to come.

- ORDER FORM -

Give the gift of *A Caregiver's Guide to Throat Cancer* to your friends, colleagues, clients, and loved ones for $19.95 each.

__YES. I want ____ copies of *A Caregiver's Guide to Throat Cancer*
__YES. I am interested in having Susan Grant speak to my organization, support group, clinic, or clients. Please contact me.

All books shipped by U.S. mail. Please include $6.00 for shipping and handling for one book, and $2.00 for each additional book. Washington State residents add 9% sales tax. For Canadian orders: please include payment in U.S. funds. Payment must accompany orders. Book orders will be processed and shipped as soon as possible.

My check or money order of $_____ is enclosed.

Please charge my: __Visa __MasterCard __American Express
Card # _____
Exp. Date _____Security Code_____
Your billing address zip code _____

Name _____
Organization _____
Address _____
City, State, Zip _____
Phone _____ Email _____

Make your check payable and mail to:
   Bella Vista Publishing
   46 Village Way, #150
   Port Ludlow, WA 98365

Got questions? Email us: info@BellaVistaPublishing.com or check out our website for the latest information as well as links for purchasing books and eBooks: www.BellaVistaPublishing.com

Made in the USA
Coppell, TX
30 January 2020